ASSESSMENT IN ADAPTED PHYSICAL EDUCATION

11045245

Judy K. Werder

**University of Minnesota
Minneapolis**

Leonard H. Kalakian

**Mankato State University
Mankato, Minnesota**

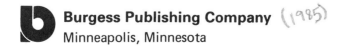
Burgess Publishing Company (1985)
Minneapolis, Minnesota

Acquisition editor: Wayne E. Schotanus
Development editor: Anne E. Heller
Copy editor: Betsey I. Rhame
Art coordinator: Judy Vicars
Composition: Edwards Brothers, Inc.
Cover design: Priscilla Heimann
Cover photograph: Cheryl Kalakian

Library of Congress Cataloging in Publication Data

Werder, Judy K.
  Assessment in adapted physical education.

  Bibliography: p.
  Includes index.
  1. Physical fitness—Testing. 2. Physical education for handicapped
children—United States. I. Kalakian, Leonard H. II. Title.
GV436.5.W47 1985   613.7'0880816   84-17436
ISBN 0-8087-3770-8

Burgess Publishing Company
7108 Ohms Lane
Minneapolis, MN 55435

Contents

Preface

This text is intended to meet a long-standing need for clarifying issues regarding the physical and motor assessment of students who are handicapped. Professionals in adapted physical education, while being committed to quality services for students, face a dilemma in the selection, administration, and interpretation of motor tests. Characterized by great variability in content, difficulty, and format of test items, motor tests are confusing at best. Unfortunately, few resources that offer clarification of these issues are available for use in training programs. Our purpose in this text is to provide a resource that assists in the development of professional motor assessment skills.

We regard assessment as the necessary link in planning instruction. Effective assessment enables the adapted physical educator to make programmatic decisions. We present motor assessment as a multifaceted process of gathering relevant information about the student. The text explains the concepts and procedures essential to each teacher's repertoire of professional assessment skills. Various methods of gathering information through precise, meaningful evaluations of students' motor strengths and needs are included throughout. From our perspective, motor assessment need not be confusing when its basic principles are applied in a systematic process of understanding each student's levels of motor functioning. The adapted physical educator who masters the principles and skills presented in the following chapters will gain credibility for the instruction planned and implemented on a daily basis.

The organization of this text has been designed to represent an accurate reflection of how assessment should be conducted in practice. Because of the heterogeneity in the ages and degrees of disabilities of children with handicaps, an understanding of these students' unique characteristics and their interaction with motor performance is the first step in initiating the assessment process.

Chapter 1 describes the unique assessment needs of students whom the adapted physical educator is likely to encounter in the assessment process. The nature of the handicapping conditions is presented to emphasize the concept that no single motor test is sufficient to determine the motor needs of such a heterogeneous population.

Chapter 2 presents a discussion of the rationale for motor assessment. Assessment, the vital link in planning instruction and in understanding the unique needs of handicapped children, represents a fulfillment of a moral obligation. Meeting the federal mandate for assessment and fulfilling the rights of handicapped children and their parents represents the legal obligation also discussed in this chapter.

Before tests can be selected and administered, the adapted physical educator should get to know the student, a process described in Chapter 3. This chapter presents procedures of inquiry that gather relevant descriptive information about a student. Because the issue of motor assessment is complex both conceptually and technically, Chapter 4 presents the questions to be asked and the guidelines to follow in judging the technical adequacy of motor test instruments. Issues of reliability and validity as they relate to assessing motor performance are discussed.

Chapter 5 demonstrates the applicability of measurement principles to the selection and administration of tests. General insights about basic types of tests and their functions are discussed. Types of psychomotor tests, procedures, and the applicability of various tests are discussed at length in Chapter 6. Specific motor tests are described with suggestions for their use in adapted physical education programs.

The final chapter in our text presents the "So what?" of the assessment process—translating assessment into action. Test scoring, interpretation of results, team planning, and individualized program planning are discussed.

The development of this text represents an effort to provide an authoritative treatise on assessment in adapted physical education. We believe that this text will become a well-used, long-lasting resource for college instructors, program supervisors, adapted physical education teachers, and others dedicated to quality physical education for *all* students.

CHAPTER 1

Who Are We Assessing?

Assessment in adapted physical education focuses on identifying the needs of students with motor difficulties and measuring the progress of students who cannot safely or successfully participate in regular mainstream physical education. Safe and successful participation in physical education without adaptations is not always a reasonable expectation for students with handicaps. Conversely, many children identified as having a handicap may not have special physical education needs. Among students with special physical education needs is a wide range of service needs, from the need for direct special instruction to the need for indirect consultation with the mainstream physical education teacher. Stein (1979, p. 6) states that "success and effectiveness of programs, activities and efforts should be based upon numbers screened out of—not screened into—special programs." He suggests that potential exists to successfully integrate 90 to 95 percent of children with handicapping conditions into regular physical education programs and activities.

Type and extent of handicap do not alone determine whether the student should be placed in regular or adapted physical education. Of great significance is the manner in which the individual copes with the condition. For example in myelomeningocele spina bifida, damage to the spinal cord (an impairment) causes dysfunction (disability) to muscles below the spina bifida site. The disability becomes a handicap only when it is identified as a factor that limits choice of life-style and pursuit of happiness. All persons with disabilities are not handicapped. Among those whose disabilities are handicapping, the handicap may present itself in a few situations only, or it may be present in most everyday situations. Furthermore, the presenting handicap may range from mild to moderate to severe.

The term *handicap* as used in this text refers to any condition that results in substantial limitations in one or more significant life activities. Such activities include language (receptive and expressive), self-care, mobility, learning, self-direction, independent living, and economic self-sufficiency.

Role of Public Law 94-142 (The Education for All Handicapped Children Act of 1975) in Determining Who We Assess

Public Law 94-142 (*Federal Register* 1977, p. 42478) states specific conditions that, when determined by assessment to be handicapping, entitle the student to federally mandated special services. All students age 3 to 21[1] who meet the P.L. 94-142 definition of handicapped and who are found through assessment to have special education needs are eligible to receive special education services. Such services, including adapted physical education services, must be made available to the student at no cost to the parent or guardian. Services must be individualized to meet the student's unique needs as identified through assessment and must be provided in the least restrictive educational environment.

Pursuant to P.L. 94-142 (*Federal Register* 1977, p. 42478), handicapped children "means those children evaluated . . . as being mentally retarded, hard of hearing, deaf, speech impaired, visually handicapped, seriously emotionally disturbed, orthopedically impaired, other health impaired, deaf-blind, multi-handicapped, or as having specific learning disabilities, who because of those impairments need special education[2] and related services."[3]

Of special significance is the phrase "who because of those impairments need special education services." This qualification renders P.L. 94-142 a double-edged sword. On the one hand, it assures that special services must be provided when necessary. On the other hand, it assures that the child is not subjected to a program that indiscriminately categorizes children on the basis of handicap label (e.g., orthopedically impaired, visually impaired, learning disabled, mentally retarded). Initially, assessment determines the type and extent of special education needs, including special physical education. Subsequently, assessment determines to what extent special needs

---

1. Specific circumstances allow each state to deviate from the 3 to 21 age range. If, for example, a state accepts as its responsibility the obligation to provide free, appropriate public education for children age 4 to 21, P.L. 94-142 requires only that the special needs of handicapped children age 4 to 21 in that state be accommodated. Under no circumstances are states mandated federally to accommodate the needs of handicapped children whose age falls outside either extreme.

2. The term *special education* means "specially designed instruction, offered at no cost to parent or guardian, to meet the unique needs of a handicapped child, including classroom instruction, instruction in physical education, home instruction, and instruction in hospitals and institutions."

3. The term *related services* means "transportation and such developmental, corrective, and other supportive services (including speech pathology and audiology, psychological services, physical and occupational therapy, recreation, and medical and counseling services, except that such medical services shall be for diagnostic and evaluation purposes only) as may be required to assist a handicapped child to benefit from special education, and includes the early identification and assessment of handicapping conditions in children."

have been met. Conditions specifically designated as handicapping by P.L. 94-142 are as follows:

I. "Deaf" means a hearing impairment so severe that the child is hindered in processing linguistic information through hearing, with or without amplification, and educational performance is thus adversely affected.

II. "Deaf-blind" means concomitant hearing and visual impairments, the combination of which causes such severe communication and other developmental and educational problems that the child cannot be accommodated in special education programs solely for deaf or blind children.

III. "Hard of hearing" means a hearing impairment, whether permanent or fluctuating, that adversely affects a child's educational performance but that is not included under the definition of "deaf" in this section.

IV. "Mentally retarded" means significantly subaverage general intellectual functioning that exists concurrently with deficits in adaptive behavior, is manifested during the developmental period, and adversely affects a child's educational performance.

V. "Multihandicapped" means concomitant impairments (e.g., mentally retarded-blind, mentally retarded-orthopedically impaired), the combination of which causes such severe educational problems that the child cannot be accommodated in special education programs designed solely for children with one of the impairments. The term does not include deaf-blind children.

VI. "Orthopedically impaired" means a severe orthopedic impairment that adversely affects a child's educational performance. The term includes impairments caused by congenital anomaly (e.g., clubfoot, absence of some member), impairments caused by disease (e.g., poliomyelitis, bone tuberculosis), and impairments from other causes (e.g., cerebral palsy, amputations, and fractures or burns that cause contractures).

VII. "Other health impaired" means limited strength, vitality, or alertness owing to chronic or acute health problems such as a heart condition, tuberculosis, rheumatic fever, nephritis, asthma, sickle cell anemia, hemophilia, epilepsy, lead poisoning, leukemia, or diabetes, which adversely affects a child's educational performance.

VIII. "Seriously emotionally disturbed" is defined as follows:

A. The term means a condition exhibiting one or more of the following characteristics over a long period of time and to a marked degree, which adversely affects educational performance:

1. An inability to learn that cannot be explained by intellectual, sensory, or health factors
2. An inability to build or maintain satisfactory interpersonal relationships with peers and teachers
3. Inappropriate types of behavior or feelings under normal circumstances

4. A general pervasive mood of unhappiness or depression
5. A tendency to develop physical symptoms or fears associated with personal or school problems.

    B. The term includes children who are schizophrenic or autistic. The term does not include children who are socially maladjusted, unless they are determined to be seriously emotionally disturbed.

  IX. "Specific learning disability" means a disorder in one or more of the basic psychological processes involved in understanding or in using language, spoken or written, that may manifest itself in an imperfect ability to listen, think, speak, read, write, spell, or do mathematical calculations. The term includes such conditions as perceptual handicaps, brain injury, minimal brain dysfunction, dyslexia, and developmental aphasia. The term does not include children who have learning problems that are primarily the result of visual, hearing, or motor handicaps; of mental retardation; or of environmental, cultural, or economic disadvantage.

   X. "Speech impaired" means a communication disorder such as stuttering, impaired articulation, a language impairment, or a voice impairment that adversely affects a child's educational performance.

  XI. "Visually handicapped" means a visual impairment that, even with correction, adversely affects a child's educational performance. The term includes both partially seeing and blind children.

Perusal of the above descriptions of each handicap category reveals that state and local interpretations are critical in determining who is eligible for P.L. 94-142 services. For example, the definition of mental retardation is couched in terms of "significantly subaverage intellectual functioning." The definition of deaf refers to any hearing impairment that "adversely affects educational performance." In each instance and in similar instances in remaining handicap categories, phrases such as "significantly subaverage" and "adversely affects" are open to interpretation. In some states, the state education agency makes such interpretations. The adapted physical education instructor must be thoroughly familiar with specific criteria that the local and state education agencies use. Such awareness assures that students eligible for P.L. 94-142 mandated services, about whom a question arises concerning safe and successful performance in physical education, are referred for assessment to determine if special physical education needs do in fact exist.

Students Needing Adapted Physical Education Who Are Not Eligible for P.L. 94-142 Services

P.L. 94-142 specifically designates those handicapping conditions that render the student eligible for special education. The law fails, however, to recognize many students who, though they do not meet the law's definition of handicapped, do have special physical education needs that cannot always be addressed in the regular mainstream curriculum. For example, among such students are those who are obese or underdeveloped, have low fitness, are awkward or clumsy, or are temporarily (acutely) handicapped. The regular physical education program is responsible for providing the necessary program modifications to accommodate the needs of such students. Physical educators must be committed to serving all children whose physical education needs cannot be met safely or successfully in the regular curriculum.

The previous discussion of "Who are we assessing?" described the wide range of characteristics of students needing developmental/adapted physical education services. Adapted physical education is indeed a cross-categorical service. There is great variance in the types of abilities and disabilities, in the severity of disabilities, in the range of physical and motor needs, and in chronological age (3 to 21 years). The tremendous heterogeneity among those who need adapted physical education demands well-trained professional staff, a wide variety of assessment methods and instruments, and comprehensive, flexible service options.

Zero Reject and Zero Fail

The question "Who are we assessing?" is not fully answered until we address the concepts of zero reject and zero fail (Eichstaedt 1976). First, virtually every student healthy enough to receive a formal education must be provided some physical education however modified. Physical educators, and especially adapted physical educators, must therefore strive to identify and meet the needs of every student for whom the school has responsibility. This is *zero reject*. Second, students should not and need not fail physical education when providers of physical education address the student's unique needs and capabilities. In this context, physical education facilitates the goal of *zero fail* by building in success.

We must be committed to identifying any student who, for whatever reason, at any given time may not be capable of safely and successfully participating in mainstream physical education. Concern for who we assess certainly includes those students guaranteed adapted physical education services through P.L. 94-142, but a commitment to human potential and the benefits of quality physical education dictates that our actions transcend mandates. The physical educator's challenge is to advocate that all students receive full opportunity for education in the physical domain in accordance with individual potential. Our responsibility as adapted physical educators is to identify the unique strengths and needs of students with handicaps and to understand the nature of such needs. Curricula and instructional strategies must then be developed to minimize the negative impact of limiting factors on achievement in physical education and to maximize the strengths of individuals.

References

Eichstaedt, C. B. Can Low Motor Skilled Children Achieve Success in Public School Physical Education? *Illinois Journal for Health, Physical Education, and Recreation* 2:11–12, 1976.

Federal Register. Final Regulations of the Education of All Handicapped Children Act, Implementation of Part B of the Education of the Handicapped Act. Department of Health, Education, and Welfare, Office of Education, Vol. 42(163), Part II, August 23, 1977, Section 121a5, Special Education, p. 42478.

Stein, J. U. The Mission and the Mandate: Physical Education, the Not So Sleeping Giant. *Education Unlimited*, June, 1979, p. 6.

CHAPTER 2

Why Are We Assessing?

When a teacher scrutinizes information derived from testing and measuring student ability or achievement, the teacher is engaging in assessment. Assessment is the critical procedure encompassing testing that renders worthwhile the time spent gathering empirical data. In assessing, one gathers descriptive information as well, and interprets the data in preparation for planning instruction. Test results by themselves do not translate into programs for students. Rather, performance evaluation and assessment of data are the seeds from which we develop a curriculum designed to meet identified needs. According to Seaman and DePauw (1982, pp. 143, 149), "Testing . . . is a data gathering technique. Assessment involves interpreting the results of measurement for the purpose of making decisions about placement, program planning, and performance objectives." Assessment, according to Bruininks (1982), is the process that improves precision in decision making.

Assessment lies at the heart of individualizing physical education for persons who have special needs. Individualized instruction (when necessary) in the least restrictive environment is the cornerstone of the Education for All Handicapped Children Act of 1975 (Public Law 94-142), and individualizing instruction is possible only when we know the individual. Assessment thus becomes the key component in fulfilling the letter and spirit of P.L. 94-142.

Does assessment necessarily occur simply because tests were administered and measurements made? Not always, according to a position taken by the American Alliance for Health, Physical Education, Recreation, and Dance[1] (1978, p. 9):

---

1. This organization was formerly called the American Alliance for Health, Physical Education, and Recreation (AAHPER). In 1980, the name was changed to reflect a growing involvement in dance. The abbreviation AAHPERD will be used for all references to the organization in this text, regardless of the actual organization name at the date of reference.

Many physical educators, special educators, and others who work with impaired, disabled or handicapped persons use tests as a drunk uses a lamppost—for support rather than illumination. Too many educators in every sphere of every discipline fail to realize that a test in itself is not important—how it is used is all that really counts. It does no good and makes no sense to administer a physical fitness test, perceptual motor scale, or developmental profile and then stick it in a drawer until next year or until the test is administered again. A testing program can be effective only when teachers . . . use results for remedial purposes, grouping, diagnosis, prescription, and to plan overall educational programs for each individual with whom they work.

Assessment is thus essential to the process of making sound decisions and planning appropriate educational programs. We emphasize assessment in adapted physical education for the many and varied reasons addressed in the remainder of this chapter.

Assessment: The Moral Obligation—the Legal Obligation

Among the principles for which any great society stands is the equal opportunity for a quality education. Simply stated, education in accordance with potential is the inalienable right of all society members.

This premise, though often preached, is not always practiced. Persons with disabilities, particularly those with special education needs, have often borne much of the brunt of educational inequity. Historically, reasons for inequities have ranged from intentional inaction to benign neglect. Advocates of full educational enfranchisement for persons with disabilities have had to lobby intensely for special legislation and have looked to the courts for assurances of educational equality.

Chronology of Advocacy

In September 1973, Congress passed legislation prohibiting discrimination based on handicapping conditions in every federally funded program or activity (Section 504 of the Rehabilitation Act of 1973, P.L. 93-112). Spurred by parent advocate groups nearly 20 years before, the Supreme Court of the United States (*Brown* v. *Board of Education,* 1954) had taken a similar stand on behalf of minority children being discriminated against in public education. The Court's statement in 1954, which was subsequently applied to the education of persons with handicaps, read as follows: "In these days it is doubtful that any child may reasonably be expected to succeed in life if he is denied the opportunity for an education. Such an opportunity where the state has undertaken to provide it, must be made available to all on equal terms."

In the wake of this decision, advocates of equality in education for the handicapped began taking their cases to court. In 1971, the Pennsylvania Association for Retarded Children (*P.A.R.C.* v. *Commonwealth of Pennsylvania*) filed suit on behalf of 13 retarded citizens in that state. Citing guarantees in the United States Constitution of due process and equal protection under the law, the suit argued that these children's access to education should be equal to that afforded other children. In a consent agreement, the court ruled in favor of the handicapped children.

The following year, the Federal Court of the District of Columbia made a similar ruling involving the full range of handicapping conditions. All children, said U.S. District Judge Joseph Waddy in the case of *Mills* v. *Board of Education*, have a right to a suitable publicly supported education, regardless of the degree of the child's mental, physical, or emotional disability or impairment. In response to arguments that this position would impose an intolerable financial burden on the community, Judge Waddy (*Mills* v. *Board of Education*) added the following: "If sufficient funds are not available to finance all of the services and programs needed and desirable in the system, then the available funds must be expended equitably in such a manner that no child is entirely excluded from a publicly supported education." In the ensuing years, an avalanche of similar suits has followed with the vast majority of judgments decided in favor of the plaintiffs.

P.L. 94-142 and Section 504

Following the 1973 Rehabilitation Act outlawing discrimination on the basis of handicap, P.L. 94-142, the Education for All Handicapped Children Act of 1975, was enacted. This nonexpiring federal legislation guarantees all handicapped students within a maximum age range of 3 to 21 years access to a free, appropriate education in the least restrictive environment.[2] The combination of P.L. 93-112, section 504, with its specific provisions for equality in education, followed by P.L. 94-142 with its guarantee of a free and appropriate education in the least restrictive environment gave persons with handicaps heretofore unprecedented educational opportunities.

Court decisions and legislation prior to P.L. 94-142 had supported overwhelmingly equal educational opportunity for all children, but such decisions and enactments did not specify how equity might be achieved. The role of assessment, though essential to the process of achieving equality, remained vague and largely implicit.

The Mandate for Assessment

P.L. 94-142 calls explicitly for assessment and delineates the course assessment must take. Pursuant to P.L. 94-142, the school district, often referred to as "the local education agency" (LEA), must affirmatively seek out children meeting the law's definition of handicapped. These children are entitled to assessment that comprehensively determines on an individual basis whether special services are necessary and what type of services are needed. The goal of P.L. 94-142 is to give each handicapped

---

2. Public Law 94-142 defines handicapped persons as those who are mentally retarded, hard of hearing, deaf, speech-impaired and language-impaired, visually impaired, seriously emotionally disturbed, orthopedically impaired, other health impaired, deaf-blind, and learning disabled. Only persons with conditions designated as handicaps are legally entitled to protection under this law.

A person may have special physical education needs (i.e., low fitness, low motor skills, environmentally deprived, obesity), but pursuant to P.L. 94-142 is neither handicapped nor entitled to special services. In such situations, the position of the AAHPERD should be invoked and the spirit of P.L. 94-142 extended. The organization position (AAHPERD 1952, p. 15) is that physical education, modified to meet individual needs, should be provided for any student "who cannot safely or successfully engage in unrestricted participation in the vigorous activities of the general physical education program."

student a free, appropriate education (individualized, if necessary) in the least restrictive environment.

Parents and children are given specific guarantees throughout the assessment process. Assessments must be administered in the child's native tongue, and the child's preferred mode of communication must be acknowledged. For example, if a deaf child relies on sign language as the primary mode of communication, the school must provide someone who can sign the test instructions. Parents are guaranteed full partnership with the school in development of their child's educational program. If parents use English as a second language, the school must provide an interpreter to assure the parents' meaningful participation. The school must not use a single assessment as the basis for determining the child's educational needs or for development of the individualized education program. Thorough, multifaceted testing, a requirement of P.L. 94-142, helps assure that the child's unique needs are understood as clearly as possible before development of an individualized program.

Tests must be used for their intended purpose only. For example, in the classroom, tests of IQ cannot be used as the basis for reading placement. Reading tests must be used for that specific purpose. In physical education, tests of motor skills cannot be used as a basis for determining physical fitness. Tests designed specifically to measure physical fitness must provide the basis for such judgments.

All assessments necessary to determine the child's educational needs are to be administered under direction of the school at no cost to the parent. Because the child is guaranteed not merely access to education but access to an *appropriate* education, assessment serves the essential purpose of determining specifically what special educational needs, if any, exist. In the event that special needs are found, the student is entitled to special services provided in the least restrictive environment.

The Mandate for Least Restrictive Environment

The term *least restrictive environment* means that students with handicaps should receive educational services in settings with "normal" students to the maximum extent possible. The term *mainstreaming* has been coined to describe education in the least restrictive environment. The least restrictive environment may be likened to a double-edged sword. One edge protects the child from being placed indiscriminately (dumped) in the mainstream. The sword's other edge protects the student from subjection to an unnecessarily restrictive, often group-paced program that arbitrarily includes other students who have also been identified as handicapped. In these latter instances, the program quality has sometimes not reflected program quality in the mainstream. In effect, the law protects the child from being educated in an environment that provides too much as well as too little restriction, and assures that the education provided is appropriate to the individual's needs. Without assessment to illuminate the handicapped student's individual strengths and needs, we cannot validly or equitably place the student at any point on the mainstream continuum.

P.L. 94-142 mandates that the education of students with handicaps be geared solely to the student's individual ability, developmental level, and needs. It rejects the historical practice of educational placement on the basis of categorical disability or label. For example, a common practice historically was to place all mentally re-tarded students in classes comprised solely of other mentally retarded students. Stu-dents were conveniently labeled and placed according to whatever special classes were available. P.L. 94-142 mandates a complete turnabout from label-generated curricula. It requires that the curricula be based on individual needs and that placement occur in the least restrictive environment regardless of labeling. Because assessment pur-suant to P.L. 94-142 identifies the student's present level of developmental and ed-ucational achievement, it spotlights what the student can do. It accentuates the pos-itive, and helps create a learning environment and curriculum characterized by positive expectations.

The individualized education program growing out of assessment must include long-range goals and short-term instructional objectives. These statements reflect spe-cific, identified needs, give direction to the student's physical education, and provide a measuring stick to assess progress. Finally, the parent and the school must agree on the focus of the student's individualized education. In the event of disagreement, P.L. 94-142 has provision for a specified due process sequence (Figure 2.1).

Performance Domains to Be Assessed

Legislators drafting P.L. 94-142 purposely included specific reference to the ne-cessity for physical education (*Federal Register* 1977, p. 42489):

> Special education as set forth in the Committee bill includes instruction in physical education, which is provided as a matter of course to all nonhandicapped children enrolled in public elementary and secondary schools. The Committee is concerned that although these services are available to and required of all children in our schools, they are often viewed as a luxury for handicapped children. The Committee expects the Commissioner of Education to take whatever action is necessary to assure that physical education services are available to all handicapped children and has specifi-cally included physical education within the definition of special education to make clear that the Committee expects such services, especially designed where necessary, to be provided as an integral part of the educational program of every handicapped child.

At this writing,[3] the definition of *special education* explicitly includes physical ed-ucation and reads as follows (*Federal Register* 1977, p. 42480): "The term special ed-ucation means specifically designed instruction, at no cost to the parent, to meet the unique needs of a handicapped child including . . . instruction in physical educa-tion." *Physical education* is further defined as "(i) the development of: (A) physical and motor fitness; (B) fundamental motor skills and patterns; (C) skills in aquatics, dance, individual and group games and sports (including intramural and lifetime sports). (ii) The term includes special physical education, adapted physical education, movement education, and motor development."

---

3. Certain modifications are currently being proposed.

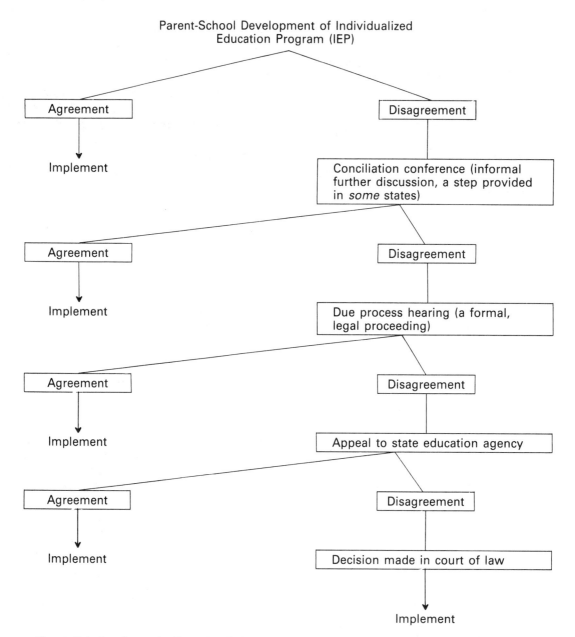

Parent-School Development of Individualized
Education Program (IEP)

Agreement

Implement

Disagreement

Conciliation conference (informal
further discussion, a step provided
in *some* states)

Agreement

Implement

Disagreement

Due process hearing (a formal,
legal proceeding)

Agreement

Implement

Disagreement

Appeal to state education agency

Agreement

Implement

Disagreement

Decision made in court of law

Implement

Figure 2.1. A schematic diagram of the due process sequence specified in P.L. 94-142 to resolve any disagreements between parents or guardians and the school.

The fact that physical education is explicitly included as part of special education testifies to the need for physical education assessment. The definition further indicates specifically what types of physical education abilities and behaviors are to be assessed.

By omission, the definition of physical education indicates what is *not* physical education. The definition makes no mention of social development, self-concept improvement, or promoting achievement in classroom studies. Such outcomes reflect the values of education through the physical. The law perceives physical education as being purely an education of the physical phenomenon. P.L. 94-142 requires that physical education address only those need areas cited in the definition. This is not to say that physical education should not be concerned with education through the physical outcomes. Historically the profession has sought to facilitate psychosocial as well as physical and motor development. Those who defined physical education in P.L. 94-142 simply chose to delimit the scope of the term. The effect of this delimitation is that assessment and subsequent development of goals and objectives for the individualized education program (IEP) must specifically address the defined components of physical education.

The Role of Assessment in Screening

Among the more important roles of assessment is the initial identification of children who appear to be having difficulty in the regular mainstream curriculum. Assessment for this purpose is termed *screening.* Screening serves the threefold purpose of (1) allaying suspicions that special needs exist, (2) initially identifying students with difficulties in physical education, and (3) being a first line of defense in assuring that special needs are identified and met early.

Screening tests, unlike more thorough diagnostic tests, require no special permission from parents or guardians to be administered (see Appendix A for examples of screening tools). Only when specific children are singled out for special testing is it necessary to attempt to secure parental permission to test.[4] Instruments generally termed screening devices are administered routinely to all members of a group. Whenever a test is routine and administered universally, no special permission to test a given student is required.

Screening specifically for early identification of problems is administered in the spirit of prevention and in the belief that early intervention is the best cure. A school district might administer a test of child development routinely to all three-year-olds. Early identification through screening, further scrutiny through diagnostic testing, and special programming may well eliminate or at least minimize the necessity for protracted, extensive special education services.

---

4. Emphasis here is on the *attempt* to secure permission. Should parents fail to respond within a prescribed, reasonable period, the school is obligated by law to proceed. Should parents refuse, the school may choose to initiate the due process sequence (Figure 2.1).

Tests used routinely to evaluate ongoing student progress in the regular main-stream curriculum may also have a screening function. A student who participated in the regular curriculum and achieved consistently at a rate well below peers should be targeted as a potential candidate for further diagnostic testing, assessment, and special services. For example, when achievement is reported in terms of percentile rank, a student who scores consistently below an established minimum may be screened from the curriculum and referred for further in-depth diagnostic assessment. Were the 25th percentile established as the minimum performance criterion and were the student to perform consistently below that criterion (i.e., below the 25th percentile on the majority of fitness battery items), that child would be targeted for diagnostic testing and assessment. Assessment could then result in an individualized curriculum and placement designed to meet the child's unique needs.

Although screening to determine who gets into adapted physical education remains an important consideration, Stein (1979, p. 6) admonishes that "success and effectiveness of programs, activities, and efforts should be based upon numbers of students screened out of—not into—special programs." He suggests that potential exists to successfully integrate 90 to 95 percent of children with handicapping conditions into regular physical education programs and activities. The concept of integration includes part-time placement in a regular program that requires direct special assistance and modifications to full-time placement in the regular mainstream without special direct assistance.

Beyond Screening—Diagnostic Testing

A student who does not achieve minimum performance standards as evidenced by screening should become a candidate for more definitive diagnostic testing. When screening confirms that performance is below standard, diagnostic testing is undertaken to identify specific areas of dysfunction. Identification of these special areas is prerequisite if specific remedial programs are to be developed.

Physical and Motor Proficiency Assessment

Perhaps the child has just failed the Kraus-Weber Test of Minimum Physical Fitness (Figure 2.2) (Kraus and Hurschland 1954). This test used as a screening device requires that all items be passed for the child to receive a score of pass on the test. Items include the following:

Item	Performance Criterion
1. Straight leg sit-up	One
2. Bent knee sit-up	One
3. Leg raise, supine position	Straight legs, feet 10 inches above surface for 10 seconds
4. Leg raise, prone position	Ten seconds
5. Trunk raise	Ten seconds
6. Toe touch	Straight legs, hold for 3 seconds

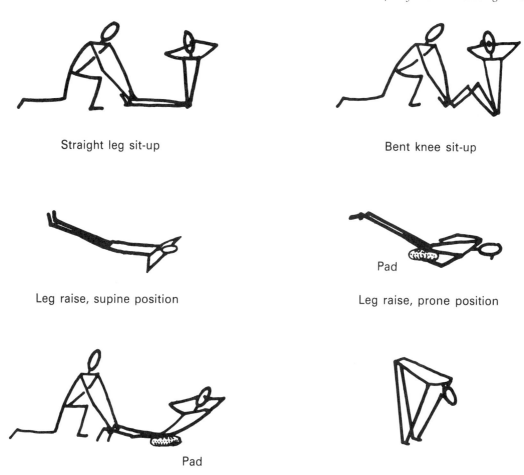

Straight leg sit-up

Bent knee sit-up

Leg raise, supine position

Pad

Leg raise, prone position

Pad

Trunk raise

Toe touch

Figure 2.2. Kraus-Weber Test of Minimum Physical Fitness (Kraus and Hurschland 1954).

As is characteristic of screening devices, the Kraus-Weber test does not measure performance (in this case, physical fitness) comprehensively. While physical fitness, including motor fitness, is comprised of approximately ten factors, the Kraus-Weber test measures but two of those factors (muscular strength and flexibility). If the child does not pass the Kraus-Weber test, the next step would be to administer a comprehensive test or tests, which would identify (i.e., diagnose) specific performance problem areas. One instrument of choice might be the American Alliance for Health, Physical Education, Recreation, and Dance Youth Fitness Test (AAHPERD 1976). Test items by component of fitness are measured as follows:

Item	Component Measured
1. Flexed arm hang (girls), pull-ups (boys)	Shoulder girdle muscular strength or endurance
2. Flexed knee sit-ups	Abdominal and hip flexor strength or endurance[5]
3. One mile or 9-minute run (chronological age 10–12 yrs); 1.5 mile or 12-minute run (CA 13 years and older)	Cardiovascular endurance
4. Shuttle run	Agility
5. Standing long jump	Explosive strength (power)
6. 50-yard dash	Speed

Note that certain physical and motor fitness components are not addressed by this test. Among these are flexibility, coordination, reaction time, and balance.[6] To be complete in the diagnosis of physical and motor proficiency, we would need to administer further tests. At this point, the teacher would select tests with items addressing components not yet covered. One such test by Fleischman (1964) measures flexibility in two ways. The Bruininks-Oseretsky Test of Motor Proficiency (Bruininks 1978) might be used to measure coordination, balance, and reaction time. Having used more than one instrument, test items representing each of the components of physical and motor proficiency will have been administered and may be supplemented by informal assessment methods.

In certain instances, students tested for physical and motor proficiency may score below entry levels of proficiency as measured by norm-referenced tests. Such tests will be limited in value because some students may function below the test's lowest percentile rank. When this occurs and no alternative is available, items appearing on a norm-referenced test may be criterion referenced or task analyzed to accommodate low functioning students. Project A.C.T.I.V.E. (Vodola 1977) exemplifies this procedure by presenting physical and motor proficiency test items in both norm-referenced and criterion-referenced formats.

Motor Skill Assessment

Attention has thus far been focused on performance assessments of physical and motor proficiency. Teachers also need to diagnose proficiency in specific motor skills

---

5. The relative fitness level of the student determines whether strength or endurance is being measured. Students able to execute only a few repetitions would be demonstrating strength, albeit limited strength. Students able to persist in a task for an extended period would be demonstrating endurance. As a rule of thumb, when the task's difficulty limits maximum repetitions to ten or less, strength is being measured. Repetitions beyond ten demonstrate muscular endurance.

6. Controversy exists over whether balance is indeed a component of motor fitness. Protagonists believe that good balance in one task is generalizable to other tasks. Antagonists allege that balance is task specific, that good balance in one task in no way assures or promotes good balance in other tasks. Should antagonists' arguments prevail, balance would lose claim to legitimacy as a motor proficiency component and test item.

(i.e., throwing, catching, kicking, striking). Here criterion-referenced instruments are helpful. These instruments characteristically break down motor skills into the sequential developmental stages that children go through in achieving mature performance. For each respective developmental stage, the instrument usually states objective performance criteria to facilitate determination of achievement. In limited respects, a criterion-referenced instrument also serves as a curriculum. If a child is at stage three in a five-stage process of learning to throw, the teacher knows from the sequenced criteria that stage four is the next sequential task to be approached.

What Assessment Does Not Do

While assessment identifies deficiencies, it does not generate labels or identify causes of deficiency. In many instances, deficiencies may be symptoms of more significant underlying causes. The purpose of assessment in adapted physical education is not, however, to determine the root causes of difficulties. If, for example, root causes are known from medical diagnosis, that information should be taken into consideration in the assessment, interpretation, and development of instructional programs. A child whose catching skills are not age appropriate may be exhibiting delayed development (symptoms) due to interference of one or more factors such as:

1. Attitudinal or environmental influences
2. Emotional or behavioral disturbances
3. Minimal neurological dysfunction (i.e., mild ataxia)
4. Delayed development of the central nervous system
5. Muscular weakness
6. Structural abnormalities

When considering factors contributing to a student's diminished performance, a team approach using allied professionals including therapists (physical, occupational, corrective), the special education teacher, the school nurse, the child's pediatrician, the behavior management specialist, and the school psychologist can prove most effective.

Interpreting Results of Assessment
to Determine Individual Needs and Educational Placement

Once diagnostic testing is completed, the assessment process is not finished. Information gathered from administration of a formal test instrument is little more than statistical data. The data gathered from informal testing and inquiry procedures complete the assessment process. Interpretations of all of these data to determine needs is what assessment is all about. (Chapter 7 gives specific guidelines for interpretation of assessment data.)

The following persons generally share in data interpretation and determine as a group the type and extent of special services needed:

1. Child's current classroom teacher
2. Special education teacher
3. Representative of the school administration
4. Child's parent or guardian
5. The child (when appropriate)
6. Other persons mutually agreed upon by the above (i.e., physical therapist, occupational therapist)

While classroom teachers are assured representation on the child's individualized planning committee, no specific reference is made to physical education teachers. However, since P.L. 94-142 includes physical education in the definition of special education and thereby designates physical education as a *primary* service, the rationale is compelling for inclusion of a physical educator on the committee. In instances of initial testing, the law does specifically indicate that someone familiar with the test and interpretation of the test results must be available. When tests have been administered and information gathered pursuant to the P.L. 94-142 definition of physical education, the physical educator is uniquely qualified to make assessments, interpret test results, and recommend remedial strategies.

Placement Alternatives

One of the major reasons for assessing is to ensure that the appropriate services are being delivered. When the planning committee has agreed on the need for a certain type of special service, it remains to determine how the child's physical education program will be delivered. P.L. 94-142 guarantees the handicapped child a physical education, specially designed when necessary, in the least restrictive environment. The law does not intend or permit indiscriminate placement in one type of service (e.g., segregated adapted physical education classes) for the child's entire physical education. For some students direct instruction in a special supplemental class may be indicated. Other students may participate fully in regular physical education classes with monitoring and assessment services only. A review of types of services (Figure 2.3) emphasizes that fewer students generally are found receiving a given service as the learning environment becomes more restrictive. This holds true for the general population since the majority of persons with disabilities are mildly disabled, and those with moderate, severe, and profound disabilities represent respectively fewer relative numbers. A more detailed discussion of placement options is presented in Chapter 7.

Assessment to Evaluate Student Progress

Progress assessments, which yield knowledge of achievement, are essential to the student, parents, and teachers. Awareness of entry-level status followed by knowl-

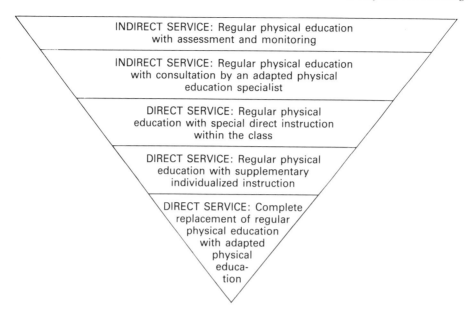

Figure 2.3. Service delivery options in adapted physical education.

edge of improvement is motivating to any student able to conceptualize the significance of improvement. When realistic goals are set and when assessment then yields evidence of progress, achievement from the child's vantage point becomes concrete. Concomitant outcomes of the student's knowledge of achievement often include heightened positive self-concept and improved motivation.

Progress assessments are essential for parents so they can know the extent of their child's achievements. Concerned parents desire the best education possible for their children, and progress assessments help parents judge improvement.

Among parents of children with disabilities, two progress-related assessment inquiries usually emerge. On the one hand, parents want to know the extent of achievement according to the child's potential. On the other hand, they desire to know the child's educational status and progress relative to peers who do not have disabilities. Finally, if parents are to assume the role of partners in their child's education, they must have a basis for determining the effectiveness of present curricula.

Teachers use progress assessments to judge curriculum effectiveness both for individual students and for the general student population. Assessing progress provides the basis for assigning grades and identifying a need for midcourse modifications in the curriculum.

Local education agencies are responsible for demonstrating to the state education agency that the P.L. 94-142 mandate is being met. Progress assessments are but one way of demonstrating program efficacy to the state education agency.

Just as local education agencies are responsible to their respective state agencies, the latter are responsible to the federal government. Assessment provides a major basis for each state's verification to the federal government that it has an affirmative plan of action to meet the P.L. 94-142 mandate, and that such plans are being implemented.

A retrospective view of this chapter suggests that the *why* of assessment cannot be separated from the *what*. *What* qualifies as a handicap? *What* is physical education? *What* are the child's special needs, and *what* alternative setting will prove least restrictive? *What* progress has been made? In the final analysis, the need to find answers to each of these questions is *why we assess*.

References

American Alliance for Health, Physical Education, Recreation, and Dance. Guiding Principles for Adapted Physical Education. *Journal of Health, Physical Education, and Recreation,* April 1952, p. 15.

——. *Testing for Impaired, Disabled, and Handicapped Individuals.* Washington, DC; The Alliance, 1975.

——. *AAHPERD Youth Fitness Test Manual.* Washington, DC: The Alliance, 1976.

Brown v. *Board of Education.* 347 U.S. 483, 74 Ct. 686, 98 L. Ed. 873, 1954.

Bruininks, R. H. Presentation delivered to Statewide Annual Leadership Conference on Adapted Physical Education. Camp Courage, Maple Lake, MN, September 23, 1982.

——. *Bruininks-Oseretsky Test of Motor Proficiency: Examiner's Manual.* Circle Pines, MN: American Guidance Service, 1978.

Federal Register. Final Regulations of the Education of All Handicapped Children Act, Implementation of Part B of the Education of the Handicapped Act. Department of Health, Education, and Welfare, Office of Education, Vol. 42(163), Part II, August 23, 1977, Section 121a14, Special Education, p. 42480.

——. Section 121a307, Physical Education, p. 42489.

Fleischman, E. A. *Examiner's Manual for the Basic Fitness Tests.* Englewood Cliffs, NJ: Prentice-Hall, 1964.

Kalakian, L. H., and Eichstaedt, C. B. *Developmental/Adapted Physical Education: Making Ability Count.* Minneapolis, MN: Burgess, 1982.

Kraus, H., and Hurschland, R. Minimum Muscular Fitness Tests in School Children. *Research Quarterly* 25(2):178, 1954.

Mills v. *Board of Education of the District of Columbia.* 348 Federal Supplement 866 (D.D.C., 1972).

Public Law 93-112, Rehabilitation Act of 1973, Section 504, Title V.

Public Law 94-142, Education for All Handicapped Children Act of 1975. 94th Congress, S.6 (20 USC 1401), November 29, 1975.

Seaman, J. A., and DePauw, K. P. *The New Adapted Physical Education: A Developmental Approach.* Palo Alto, CA: Mayfield, 1982.

Stein, J. U. The Mission and the Mandate: Physical Education, the Not So Sleeping Giant. *Education Unlimited,* June 1979, p. 6.

Vodola, T., Director. Project A.C.T.I.V.E. Grant sponsored by Elementary and Secondary Education Act, Title III-IV(c) and Division of Research, Planning, and Evaluation, New Jersey State Department of Education, 1977.

CHAPTER 3

Getting to Know the Student

The motor skill proficiency demonstrated by a student today has been shaped by events that make up his or her history of growth and development. In the motor domain, assessing a child's current level of motor performance is not enough. The physical educator conducting a comprehensive assessment must also understand what has shaped that current performance. Deleterious events, physical and sensory impairments, and environmental deprivation as well as many other historical factors affect a child's current motor skill functioning. Upon receiving a referral for developmental/adapted physical education, the tester should become a "detective" who gathers relevant historical as well as current information to better understand and plan for the student's educational program.

Medical Records

To plan an appropriate physical education program for a child who is handicapped, the educator must check health and medical records for relevant information. In the school, the nurse or other health personnel can assist in reviewing the school's health records for a particular student. Health files should be examined for essential information including

1. Chronic or acute illnesses (e.g., diabetes, chronic heart ailment, chronic asthma)
2. Physical impairments (e.g., cerebral palsy, muscular dystrophy, amputee)
3. Sensory impairments (e.g., loss of vision or hearing, speech or language difficulties)
4. Records of mild illnesses (e.g., frequent colds, headaches, stomachaches) and records of absenteeism due to illness

5.   Names of physicians and therapists
6.   Phone numbers of parents for emergency situations
7.   Medications and their purposes

The quick perusal of a student's health file can be a valuable expenditure of time, revealing vital historical information about the health history.

This preliminary examination of a child's history may pinpoint sources for more in-depth assessment. For example, a school health file indicates that Amy gets physical therapy once a week. It is crucial for the developmental/adapted physical educator to learn the reasons for and the nature of the therapy. Such information helps the teacher design and develop appropriate activities for the developmental/adapted physical education program that will not contradict the goals of the therapy.

Before obtaining information from a therapist or a physician, it is important to follow due process procedures and secure parental permission for the doctor or therapist to release and discuss information. The records and opinions of physicians can provide important data. For example, if a student has a diagnosis of severe juvenile rheumatoid arthritis, an exchange of information among parent, doctor, and teacher is vital. Giving the physician information about educational planning to meet individual needs is just as important as gathering data from the medical doctor. Physicians and school personnel must work cooperatively to plan an appropriate physical education program for a child who is handicapped. Figure 3.1 presents a sample form that can be used to assist in gathering relevant information from doctors. Relevant historical data may include the following:

1.   Medical diagnosis
2.   Severity and prognosis
3.   Symptoms relevant to a physical education setting
4.   Past and current course of treatment
5.   Restricted activities
6.   Telephone numbers and addresses of relevant medical personnel
7.   Any recommendations for physical activity made by the physician

Once again we emphasize that parental permission must be secured before gathering historical medical information.

School Files

Another potentially valuable source of information that can contribute to a comprehensive developmental/adapted physical education assessment is the student's cumulative school file. The "home room" teacher and the school guidance counselor have access to a cumulative file for each student assigned to them. These files are established for each student when he or she enters school, and the files "follow" the

MEDICAL AUTHORIZATION FORM
LONG-TERM DISABILITY

REGION 11E

DATE SENT: _____ Minnesota Developmental/Adapted Physical Education

Minnesota State Law requires that all students participate in physical education on a regular basis. If a permanent or long-term disability interferes with participation in the regular physical education program, an individualized physical education curriculum will be planned around the student's motor strengths and abilities. The student shall be enrolled in the adapted program based on completion of this form.

Student's Name _____ D.O.B. _____ School _____ Grade _____

Parent/Guardian _____ Phone _____

Disability _____

_____

Expected Duration of Disability _____

Medication (implication for physical activity) _____

_____

The following activities will be adapted to the student's individual capabilities. Please check any activity you would NOT recommend for the above student.

I. Physical Fitness Activities
___arm-shoulder strength
___abdominal strength
___flexibility (range of motion)
___cardio-respiratory endurance
___leg strength

II. Locomotor Activities
___creeping
___crawling
___walking
___running
___sliding
___hopping
___jumping
___skipping
___galloping

III. Non-Locomotor Activities
___bending   ___hanging
___twisting   ___balancing
___pushing   ___swinging
___pulling
___lifting

IV. Aquatics
___swimming skills
___water play
___diving

V. Object Control Skills
___catching
___kicking
___striking
___overhand throwing
___underhand throwing
___ball bouncing

VI. Other Activities not Recommended:
_____
_____
_____
_____
_____
_____
_____
_____
_____
_____

COMMENTS: _____

_____

Your input will assist us in determining an appropriate instructional program.

Date: _____   Signed: _____, M.D.

Phone Number: _____

Figure 3.1. Sample medical information form. (Minnesota Developmental/Adapted Physical Education, Region 11E, 1981)

student through school until graduation. Cumulative files generally contain objective information such as

1. Student's name and address
2. Names and addresses of parents or guardians
3. Family status (siblings and ages)
4. Emergency contact persons
5. Standardized achievement test scores
6. General school progress reports
7. Schoolwork samples (sometimes)
8. Photograph of the student

The content of cumulative records varies from school district to school district. There has been some effort recently to remove all subjective reports and to include only objective information. Upon referral of a handicapped student for motor assessment, the tester should immediately examine the student's cumulative file to obtain the preliminary information previously listed.

Another source of historical information available in the school is the "special education file." For every student who has been determined to be handicapped according to P.L. 94-142, a special education record should be on file. The special education file can provide a wealth of important historical information such as

1. Primary disability and when determined
2. Severity of disability (level of special education services provided in the past)
3. All special education services provided currently and in the past, and names of service providers
4. Assessment information from previous special education assessments
5. Previous individualized education programs (IEPs)
6. Records of progress toward IEP objectives
7. All due process forms and permission forms

This special education information can be extremely valuable to the developmental/adapted physical education assessment. For example, a history of distraction and severe learning disability can guide the tester when deciding what types of motor tests to administer. This information will help school personnel choose the most appropriate tests to administer to a student who is highly distractible and has receptive language difficulties. Finding out which special education teachers have worked previously with the student provides yet another avenue for gathering relevant information.

Insights From Parents

Parents have the right to be involved in developing the assessment process for their child, and can be involved in various ways besides those required by P.L. 94-142. They can play an essential role in the assessment process by reporting information about their child's history. Once a student is referred for developmental/adapted physical education assessment, parents should be contacted to provide needed information about the student's developmental history by being interviewed or by completing case histories. Often such information is available only from parents, since school personnel have little or no knowledge of the student's past and do not usually observe the student's movement behaviors outside the school setting. Figure 3.2 suggests a useful format for interviewing parents about their child's motor development history. To be an effective means of gathering historical information, an interview should be sensitive and efficient. The interviewer encourages the parents to talk freely, while limiting his or her own participation. The purpose of the interview should be made clear to the parents: to gather information about their child's motor development history. Interview questions reflect this purpose and are factual in nature, for example, "At what age did Johnny begin to walk?" Besides providing insights about the child's motor development history, parents can also share observations about the child's behavior while playing and interacting with peers and family members.

Insights From Other School Personnel

Other sources of valuable historical information about a child's development are other teachers in the school. Previous classroom teachers, speech clinicians, special education teachers, and physical education teachers may be able to share observations about a student's motor development, fitness, and play behavior. This historical information should if possible be compiled cumulatively in chronological order to reveal the child's general patterns of growth and motor development. Historical information from school personnel can be obtained by interviews or by the use of other informal measures such as rating scales or checklists. Other school personnel who may be able to provide relevant historical insights are nurses, administrators, teacher aides, or occupational and physical therapists. The school nurse might share information that is not available in the student's school health file. Often the school nurse will have had meetings or conversations with parents, physicians, or therapists. Although the essential information is usually documented in the health file, insights, opinions, and judgments of school personnel should not be ignored, but should be weighed with other informal assessment information.

Who Assesses What?

The assessment of the motor functioning of handicapped children is not always conducted by developmental/adapted physical education teachers. Motor assessment may be conducted by mainstream physical education teachers, developmental/adapted physical education specialists, occupational therapists, physical therapists, corrective therapists, classroom teachers, special education teachers, and sometimes by psy-

Parent Interview
Adapted Physical Education
Gross Motor Development

Student _____

Interview Date _____

Date of Birth _____ Grade/Teacher _____

Interviewer _____

Name of Parent/Guardian _____

Address _____ Phone _____

_____

_____

_____ :

(Child's Name)

	YES	NO	UNSURE
A. Motor Development			
1. First walked without crawling beforehand (creeping on hands and knees)			
2. First walked before 12 months			
3. First walked between 12–18 months			
4. First walked between 18–24 months			
5. First walked after 24 months			
6. Seemed to sit, stand, and walk late			
7. Walks on toes			
8. Walks flat-footed			
B. Coordination			
9. Falls frequently			
10. Bumps into things, people frequently			
11. Loses balance easily			
12. Seems to show shaky, jerky movements			
C. Body Awareness			
13. Feels uncomfortable about his or her body			
14. Confused easily about directions (e.g., right, left, forward, sideways)			
15. Understands basic body parts and their relationships (e.g., front, back, arm, foot)			
D. Physical Fitness			
16. Tires easily			
17. Overweight			
18. Seems to lack strength			
19. Lacks vitality (energy, enthusiasm)			
E. Social and Emotional Development			
20. Enjoys balls, bats, and other movement toys (jump ropes, rebounder)			
21. Plays outdoors often			
22. Plays vigorously with other children			
23. Enjoys gym class			
24. Participates in extracurricular physical activities			
25. Enjoys playing physical games and sports			

Figure 3.2. Suggested format for interviewing parents or guardians about the child's motor development history.

chologists. The person conducting the motor assessment should be thoroughly familiar with the test content and procedures. Most desirable is for a physical education teacher, a developmental/adapted physical education specialist, or a therapist to conduct the motor assessment.

Assessment by the Physical Educator

Physical education teachers are involved in assessment at a variety of levels. The elementary physical education teacher may be responsible for conducting initial screening at preschool or kindergarten-age levels. Screening is a type of general assessment administered to all students in a class. At early age levels, motor screening becomes part of a larger, more comprehensive screening of general cognitive, affective, and psychomotor development. Children diagnosed as having problems at early age levels are usually referred for more in-depth diagnostic assessment.

Physical education teachers also conduct physical education screening tests at other elementary grade levels. General physical fitness tests, like the AAHPERD Youth Fitness Test, are often administered at intermediate and secondary grade levels. The Youth Fitness Test, while generally not used for developmental/adapted physical education screening, is used to determine students' overall levels of physical fitness as compared to a norm group. Overall fitness data can tell the teacher how each class compares with a national average in the fitness subtest areas. Teachers can subsequently make decisions and plan their instruction around areas of strength and weakness.

At junior and senior high school levels, physical educators may administer tests corresponding to certain curricular units of instruction. For example, a teacher may select a soccer skills test at the end of a soccer unit. In a skills test, students are asked to demonstrate their proficiencies in specific skills presented during the physical education class. Secondary level physical educators may also administer group fitness tests, and sometimes they may elect to test students' knowledge of physical education concepts with a written test.

Today most physical education curricula are objective-based with clearly defined criteria for each grade level. Objective-based curricula readily lend themselves to ongoing criterion-referenced assessment. In some schools, physical education teachers must report their classes' percentage of mastery on curricular objectives taught during the school year. Objective-based programs with curriculum-imbedded assessment provide a clearly defined system for program planning, individualizing instruction, and monitoring pupil progress toward objectives. Objective-based instruction has had a tremendous impact on physical education. Curriculum planning, accountability, and curriculum-imbedded assessment are now integral parts of a field in which individualization had seemed to some to be next to impossible.

Regular physical educators and developmental/adapted physical educators have recently been faced with the challenge of conducting diagnostic testing. Assessing for diagnosis requires the teacher to gather data that help diagnose the specific characteristics of a student's motor difficulties. Diagnostic motor testing attempts to pinpoint particular problem areas of motor development such as balance or eye-hand coordination. In-depth assessment of motor functioning is usually administered individually, and diagnostic tests are usually formal tests, although informal criterion-referenced tests may also be used. Formal diagnostic tests are usually administered in one test session. In contrast, criterion-referenced tests may be cumbersome and more time-consuming for assessment in each objective area. Because diagnostic tests are generally administered to students individually, it is difficult for the regular physical education teacher to find the time to test children. In some school districts, time is allotted in the physical educator's schedule to conduct such assessments. In other districts, developmental/adapted physical educators assume responsibility for all individual physical education assessments.

The content of tests administered by physical educators can vary and may include tests of sports skills, fundamental locomotor patterns, or perceptual-motor abilities. The content of these tests should be directly related to the skills taught in the physical education curriculum. When selecting tests, physical educators must thoroughly examine content to determine whether the test assesses skills important in physical education.

Assessment by Therapists

In recent years, occupational therapists (OTs) and physical therapists (PTs) have undertaken new contributing roles in public schools. P.L. 94-142 mandates the provision of therapies as related services when determined necessary to a handicapped student's special education. When therapists are members of the child study team, portions of motor assessment can be conducted by the occupational therapist or the physical therapist. Traditionally therapists function from a medical model, and physical educators operate within an educational model. Physical education teachers primarily assess observable, measurable motor *skills*, while therapists tend to assess the *processes* underlying movement. Therapists, like physical educators, conduct both formal and informal assessment, depending on the purpose of the assessment.

Occupational therapists in the schools might administer formal or informal tests to identify the handicapped student's functional performance levels in the following areas (Gilfoyle 1981):

1. Gross and fine motor skills
2. Reflex and reaction development
3. Developmental landmarks
4. Sensorimotor functioning
5. Neuromuscular functioning
6. Self-help skills
7. Prevocational skills
8. Social interaction skills

Several areas of assessment overlap with physical education (gross motor skills) and with special education assessment (self-help skills, prevocational skills, and social interaction skills). This sort of overlap of professional responsibilities has been the subject of some controversy. Therapists and educators can, however, work cooperatively to plan a comprehensive assessment process that avoids duplication and yet prevents gaps in assessment. Upon receiving and reviewing the referral of a handicapped student for motor assessment, it is vital for physical educators and therapists to plan and decide who will conduct which type of assessment. Each professional has unique, relevant information to bring to the team meeting. The interdisciplinary approach to assessment emphasizes sharing, respecting, and learning from each team member's contribution.

In some schools, physical therapists are available to assist in motor assessment. For students who are physically handicapped, like those with cerebral palsy, motor assessment is based primarily on a medical model. Evaluation conducted by a physical therapist can provide valuable insights for planning appropriate physical activities. Physical therapists can evaluate tonus, range of motion, posture patterns, and patterns of movement of physically handicapped students. Results of a clinical evaluation of motor functioning by a physical therapist are then combined with information gathered by the physical educator. In cases of physically handicapping conditions when only early diagnostic information is available, a current evaluation by a physical therapist may shed light on present functional capacity and subsequent implications for physical education programming. In addition to identifying physiological (motor), topographical (affected parts of the body), and etiological (causative) factors used in classifying physical handicaps, physical therapists can also conduct supplemental evaluations including

1. Physical status (growth, developmental level, bone age)
2. Posture evaluation
3. Eye-hand behavior patterns (eye dominance, eye movements, fixation, convergence, grasp)
4. Visual status (sensory defects, motor defects)
5. Early reflexes
6. Range of joints and strength
7. Levels of motor skills (locomotor, head control, trunk control)
8. Motor symptoms (spasticity, athetosis, ataxia, rigidity, tremors)

Although physical therapists can provide information vital to the physical educator, intervention becomes the point of departure for the two disciplines. The therapist and the educator's challenge is to translate relevant evaluative information into appropriate educational goals and objectives for each physically handicapped student. The objectives defined for the student must be observable, measurable motor *skills* that are activity-based within the educational model (rather than therapeutic goals within the medical model, which are more appropriately provided in a clinical setting).

References

Gilfoyle, E. M. *Training: Occupational Therapy Educational Management in Schools (TOTEMS).* Washington, DC: U.S. Office of Special Education and Rehabilitative Services, 1981.

CHAPTER 4

Can the
Measurement Be Trusted?

Data derived from testing children with disabilities provide the basis for identifying special physical education needs and subsequent development of individualized education programs. Data derived from testing also provide the basis for determining how effective the individualized education has been. Interpretation of such data is important to teachers, parents, and children. Teachers need to judge program efficacy. Parents need to know how well their child is doing compared with other, similar children (i.e., "In what percentile is my child?"), and to know how their child's abilities compare with developmentally sequenced performance criteria for all children. Parents also often want to know how their child with a handicap is doing compared with children who are not handicapped. Lastly, interpretation of such data is also important to any child who understands progress, since knowledge of progress is essential in maintaining learner motivation.

Given the pervasive significance of accurate test data and the interpretation of data in identifying and meeting the needs of children with handicaps, it is essential that we make judgments about the quality of the data base from which assessment evolves. An expression from computer science is applicable to administering and interpreting tests. The admonition "garbage in, garbage out" speaks graphically to the reality that all tests yield data. When the data are of questionable integrity, however, but are nevertheless used to make educational decisions, can those decisions be of value? We should not have faith simplistically in a given test whether it be published and allegedly standardized or teacher-made. Even when we have judged a test satisfactory for a given purpose, we must remain aware of factors extrinsic to the instrument that can affect the quality of our information. When determining the trustworthiness of test data, scholarly scrutiny should be the rule, and the following considerations are in order.

Validity

If a test measures what it alleges to measure, that test is said to be *valid*. Among persons new to testing, this concept may seem so basic as to scarcely warrant mention. Perhaps because the concept of validity seems simplistic, concern for validity by both test developers and test users is sometimes inadequate. The following are cases in point.

Content Validity.   Content validity refers to the appropriateness of the test items for measuring motor performance and for sampling the motor domain. Tests of physical and motor proficiency are said to be valid to the extent that sufficient representative components of physical and motor proficiency are included and assigned appropriate weight in the battery. For example, assume that physical and motor proficiency is comprised of ten mutually exclusive items as follows (Kalakian and Eichstaedt 1982):

Physical Fitness
1. Muscular strength
2. Muscular endurance
3. Flexibility
4. Cardiovascular endurance

Motor Fitness
5. Balance
6. Speed
7. Reaction time
8. Coordination
9. Agility
10. Explosive strength (combination of speed and strength)

Now assume (as is often the case) that a given test of physical and motor proficiency is comprised of fewer than ten items. We might well assume that some components of fitness are not being tested, and that the teacher will not know the child's prowess in components not addressed. If the child is proficient in components of fitness not measured and happens to be deficient in components measured, the child will be judged less fit than she or he really is. If the child is proficient in items measured but deficient in items not measured, the child is likely to be judged more fit than he or she really is. In either instance, the validity of the data is questionable, because the test purporting to measure physical and motor proficiency is not comprehensive. For the teacher using this test battery, a suggested solution would be to include items from other tests that address proficiencies not covered by the first test, or to administer a similar test to examine congruent validity.

Some items lack content validity because the criterion for success is questionable. Consider tests of throwing accuracy that use a target configuration other than concentric circles. One test (Vodola 1976), standardized for use with persons who have disabilities, has a target composed of concentric rectangles (Figure 4.1). Note that an accuracy deviation in the 3 or 9 o'clock directions is less severely penalized than de-

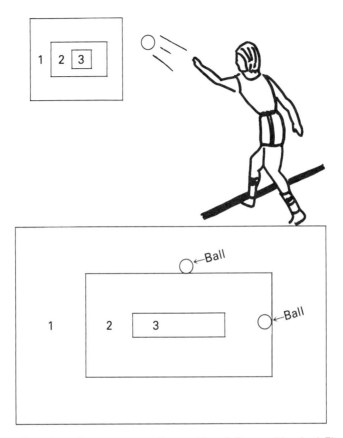

Figure 4.1. Item testing throwing accuracy, Township of Ocean Physical Fitness Test (Vodola 1977). Both balls are equidistant from the target center, yet one throw is awarded two points (3 o'clock) and the other is awarded one point (1 o'clock).

viations in the 12 and 6 o'clock directions. The test user must ask if this specific procedure has been prescribed for some reason, or if the test developer has erred in the attempt to measure accuracy.

Construct Validity. A test is said to lack *construct validity* if the test is not representative of the domain of motor performance it claims to represent. An effective test is solidly based on motor development research and theory. Among available motor tests are some that are technically inadequate as well as lacking predictive validity. A valid motor test should yield predictions that can be assessed in the physical education class.

Tests subjected to the statistical procedure of factor analysis during their construction are generally relatively complete in their coverage of components. Factor analysis helps test developers to identify battery items that do not correlate with each other. When item scores do not correlate, this indicates that different proficiencies are being measured. If a sufficiently wide variety of potential battery items is subjected to factor analysis, the forthcoming battery will probably present items that represent and properly weight all fitness components.

One test exemplifying incomplete coverage of components is the Special Fitness Test for the Mildly Mentally Retarded (AAHPERD 1976), which includes the following items:

1. Flexed-arm hang (muscular strength and endurance)
2. Sit-ups (muscular strength and endurance)
3. Shuttle run (agility)
4. Softball throw (coordination and perhaps upper extremity explosive strength)
5. Standing long jump (lower extremity explosive strength)
6. 50-yard dash (speed)
7. 600-yard run-walk (cardiovascular endurance)

While certain of these items are in themselves of questionable validity for reasons that will be discussed later, the important point to note here is that the test does not address three fitness components generally considered part of the physical and motor proficiency domain (balance, flexibility, and reaction time). The tester's task would be to locate test items to measure each of the otherwise unmeasured components in the battery.

The validity of any given test item is questionable if that item is measuring more than one proficiency. In such instances, the tester cannot ascertain the intervening factors of a performance deficiency. For example, a score in the 50-yard dash, allegedly a measure of speed, is confounded by the additional requirements of reaction time and explosive strength. Does a slow 50-yard dash time indicate poor speed, slow reaction time, weak explosive strength, or some combination of the three (Figure 4.2)? In this instance, what valid interpretation can the teacher make of such data? One solution is to specify a flying start, thereby minimizing the contributions of reaction time and explosive strength to the student's elapsed time. Remember, however, that if norms are being used, test items must be administered exactly as specified in the test manual. The tester must follow administration instructions precisely. Any deviation compromises the instrument's validity. If instructions for administering an item specifically state "do not demonstrate," under no circumstances may the tester demonstrate. If the test calls for three trials with the best of three serving as the score, three trials, no more and no less, must be administered. Errors of this type are often committed unintentionally because the tester is not thoroughly familiar with the battery items. A good rule for testers is to know the test administration procedures so well that the manual need be referred to only briefly and occasionally in the student's presence.

In some instances, tests are accompanied by formal examiner instructions. After studying these, the reader is usually tested on pertinent information. If the reader achieves a passing score according to the test developer's criteria, the reader is then judged a competent administrator of the test.

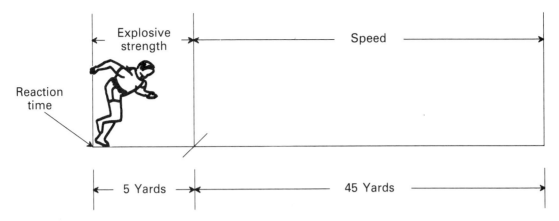

Figure 4.2. Does the 50-yard dash measure speed alone, or is speed measurement complicated by inclusion of related proficiencies such as reaction time and explosive strength?

To be valid, a test must address the presenting problem. Just as a test of intelligence cannot validly serve as a basis for reading level placement (a test specifically designed to measure reading ability must be used), so tests of motor skills cannot validly serve as a basis for evaluating physical fitness. To be valid, a test must be used specifically for the purpose for which it was intended.

Factors Influencing Validity.   The child's disposition at test time can affect validity. Some children tire easily and may not demonstrate proficiency according to potential if tested late in the day or after a particularly trying day. Some children may be under the influence of medication, which may affect motor performance, or they may be in the process of having medications or dosages changed. In some cases, performance may be affected because the child did not take prescribed medication.

Some tests rely on the element of competition to evoke the best responses from children. Some children, particularly some with disabilities, may not relate well to competition and may find themselves at an inherent disadvantage. Others, particularly those with information-processing deficits (i.e., mentally or emotionally handicapped), may not see the significance of trying to do their best. In such instances, strong extrinsic motivators-reinforcers may be necessary to evoke the best responses.

Many persons, particularly those with limited abilities relative to the proficiencies tested, exhibit relatively short attention spans. The examiner should remain observant and sensitive to shifts in attention, recognizing that such shifts will lower the performance level. In such instances, the tester must seek new ways to attract and motivate the student, or abandon testing altogether for the time being.

When determining appropriateness of a test for any given individual, the tester must be aware of the population for which the test was intended. Was the test being administered to a blind student normed with blind peers? Should severely retarded students be subjected to norms developed for persons moderately retarded? Were persons from your student's locality included in the development of norms? Ideally, when norms are applied, the student should be compared with peers. The tester is otherwise confronted with having to compare apples and oranges. Since regional differences in performance sometimes affect norms (Espenschade and Eckert 1980), norms should be drawn from large, representative samples of peers. Sometimes test developers have been forced to rely on less than optimum sample sizes when compiling norms for persons with handicaps. Whenever possible, the tester should note the number of persons by age and sex for each test item to determine the representativeness of norms. When the number in a normative group is small from one age group to the next for any given test item, the evaluator often observes a phenomenon called "spiking norms." Figure 4.3, an excerpt from the *Motor Fitness Testing Manual for the Moderately Retarded,* is an example of spiking norms resulting from inadequate sample size (AAHPERD 1976).

Another concern when applying norms to one's students is that the norms discriminate among different levels of proficiency. If norms are not challenging and if everyone exceeds the 90th percentile, or if norms are so challenging that no one exceeds the 10th percentile, what basis does the teacher have for determining relative

Long Jump—Males (Measured in Inches)
70th Percentile

CA =	6	7	8	9	10	11	12	13	14	15	16
N =	10	25	40	46	47	52	69	59	73	48	52

Figure 4.3. Example of spiking norms (*Motor Fitness Testing Manual for the Moderately Retarded,* AAHPERD 1976). (CA = chronological age; N = number in sample)

abilities? The applied norms must be sensitive to the varying abilities of those tested.

Validity can be affected whenever the student's disability interferes unnecessarily with completion of the task. For example, an agility run requiring the student to shuttle between lines 30 feet apart, including picking up and depositing blocks, will not yield valid agility data among blind students. Instead, a four-count squat-thrust (burpee) may provide a more valid measure of rapid direction-change ability, because locomotion through visual space and object manipulation are not required.

Among mentally retarded children, agility-run results have been correlated significantly with mental age (Speakman 1977). The effect is that, among mentally handicapped persons, higher mental age is associated with faster agility-run times. Agility runs among mentally handicapped students are therefore probably not a good measure of agility and are at best a poor test of mental age. The student's mental retardation limits the ability to understand task demands, making the test validity doubtful.

Children must comprehend what is being asked of them. Tests in the psychomotor domain should not become inadvertent measures of language comprehension. When in doubt, it is sometimes appropriate to ask the child to relate the tester's instructions in her or his own words.

Some children with special needs who are nonverbal or who are just becoming verbal may have vocabularies that limit their ability to process verbal information. The tester should then try to identify key words or terms to communicate the behavior desired. In this way, the critical words are not obscured by the less important. An example of this technique is found in *I CAN* program assessment procedures, wherein specific "action words" are identified and recommended by the test developer (Wessel 1976).

In considering the child's level of language development, the teacher should be cognizant of both expressive and receptive language abilities. *Expressive language* refers to language that the child speaks. *Receptive language* refers to language that the child hears and comprehends. Among children with special needs who also manifest language delays, receptive language development often exceeds expressive language. The tester may also deal with children for whom English is a second language. Concern for validity then demands that instructions be given in the child's native tongue.

For some children with hearing impairments, signing and finger spelling are the preferred communication mode. Signs and finger spelling must then form the basis for communicating test instructions. When hard-of-hearing children do rely in part or in full on speech reading, the examiner when speaking must always face the student. The examiner's speech patterns should not be altered, and when possible the student's back should be facing the sun or any bright lights. Note also that the lips of persons sporting moustaches or beards are particularly problematic for persons who must read speech.

In test-retest or pretest-posttest situations, the teacher should be certain that test conditions during the second administration are identical to those during the first administration. Is the time of day similar? Are weather conditions similar? If the child uses a brace or assistive device for ambulation, was such a device (even more specifically, the same device) used during the first test? Is a wheelchair ambulator using the same or at least the same quality chair, and has chair maintenance improved or deteriorated during the ensuing time? These are but a few examples of the many factors that can influence the outcome of a test. Unless such factors are eliminated or at least considered, comparison of pretest and posttest results may be invalid or only partially valid.

These are only some of the factors affecting the validity of tests and test items administered in an adapted physical education setting. The foregoing considerations should not be perceived as exhaustive. They are examples intended to heighten sensitivity to the kinds of factors that can affect test validity, and hence the degree to which a measurement can be trusted.

Reliability

Reliability addresses the concern for consistency. A test is deemed *reliable* if repeated measures, under substantially similar conditions, yield consistent results. For example, a scale is called reliable if the same poundage registers each time a given mass is weighed. In measuring human performance, however, one seldom expects or achieves such precision. It should suffice if the tester is satisfied that an observed proficiency is representative of the student's true capability.

In administering a test item that requires more than one trial (i.e., add the total of three trials or score the best of three trials), one should observe the consistency of the student's performances. Consistency would tend to support reliability, and the tester should be concerned when the quality of performance among trials seems erratic.

In developing one's own test of some psychomotor skill, say throwing for accuracy, the tester would want to determine the quantity of throws necessary for throwing performance to stabilize. Throws executed prior to the achievement of performance repeatability should be considered unreliable for measurement purposes and be used only as warm-up (AAHPERD 1976). A counter argument to this approach is the observation that too many trials may yield some learning effect. The alternative, however, the acceptance of unreliable data, seems the greater evil.

Objectivity, an important aspect of reliability, addresses the concern for repeatability. We have discussed the consistency of one examiner's scoring. Objectivity addresses scoring consistency between examiners. Testers who are scoring in quantifiable measures have the edge on testers scoring repeatability. For example, we expect greater reliability between examiners when they count sit-ups than when they judge Special Olympics floor exercise contestants. Indeed, in many instances objectively quantifiable data simply cannot be derived from the performance or behavior observed. A significant factor affecting the objectivity of results, whether they be of the stopwatch (objective) or rating scale (subjective) type, is rapport between examiner and student. For whatever reasons, sex of the examiner and age of the examiner versus age of the student may be factors influencing student performance. To some students, one teacher's demeanor may appear to be more threatening than another's. Results can be affected by the presence of others during the test, and results may be further affected by whether the others in attendance are parents, siblings, peers, authority figures, or strangers. Any combination of the above circumstances can cause one tester to elicit a student performance significantly different from that elicited by another tester. This reliability is reported in some test manuals and can be calculated easily.

Items that yield quantifiable scores (i.e., number of pull-ups, pulse, flexed-arm-hang time) tend to be relatively more reliable than those items yielding rating scale scores (i.e., always, sometimes, never). Assignment of rating scale scores tends to be relatively more dependent on the subjective opinion of the rater. Whenever rating scales provide the basis for gathering data, concern for reliability dictates that rating criteria be stated as objectively as possible, preferably in behavioral terms. In such cases, calculating interrater agreement can assure acceptable reliability.

Reliability is thus a critical concern when any informal assessment methods are used. When observing and assessing a student's motor performance, calculating the interrater reliability of the assessment method is important. Interrater reliability can be readily calculated when more than one person observes and scores a student's movement by working out the "percent of agreement":

$$\frac{\text{Agreements}}{\text{Agreements} + \text{Disagreements}} \times 100 = \% \text{ Agreement}$$

The assessment is considered adequate if the interrater reliability is at least 80 percent.

Reliability is of particular significance whenever one person's test results are to be interpreted by another person. If the person interpreting the data might have assigned scores different from those with which he or she is working, then an individualized education program based on those different scores would probably take on a different emphasis. These circumstances render the test reliability questionable, thus making the test validity questionable.

Reliability and validity are interrelated because we cannot achieve validity without having first achieved reliability. A test is not reliable unless it yields consistent and representative behaviors. If the data are not representative of the student's true abilities, then the test is not measuring what it purports to measure and cannot be valid.

While validity is not possible without reliability, reliability is possible without validity. For example, if a tester were to measure balance by repeated correct foot placements on a 4-inch-wide stripe painted on the floor, a quantifiable score would result. If more than one performance yielded consistent scores, the tester might suspect that the task was reliable. Given these data, students could be ranked according to ability. Now assume that the task is repeated, only the floor stripe is replaced by a 4-inch-wide beam placed 2 feet above the ground. If the rankings following performance on the elevated beam are different, could both items have measured the same ability? Perhaps, while performance on the relatively less threatening stripe measured balance, performance on the relatively more threatening elevated beam measured courage in addition to balance. The latter item may have yielded reliable information, but interpretation of the data in terms of balance would render validity suspect. An item, even though reliable, must not therefore be considered automatically valid.

When Tests Are Less Than Perfect

No test is perfect, and no testing environment is ever completely right. At best we strive for tests and conditions somewhere between less than perfect and more than adequate. Achievement of that goal is facilitated when the teacher assumes the role of both detective and scholar. Recognizing that some tests are indeed technically inadequate and that testing environments are sometimes not conducive to eliciting best responses, the teacher is compelled to rely on her or his professional judgment. By understanding the factors that limit the trustworthiness of test data, we take an important first step in minimizing the potential negative impact of such factors on important assessment functions.

References

AAHPERD. *Motor Fitness Testing Manual for the Moderately Mentally Retarded.* Washington, DC: The Alliance, 1976.

AAHPERD. *Special Fitness Test for the Mildly Mentally Retarded.* Washington, DC: The Alliance, 1976.

Espenschade, A., and Eckert, H. *Motor Development.* Columbus, OH: Charles E. Merrill, 1980.

Kalakian, L. H., and Eichstaedt, C. B. *Developmental/Adapted Physical Education: Making Ability Count.* Minneapolis, MN: Burgess, 1982.

Speakman, H. G. B. A Motor Fitness Test Suitable for Trainable Mentally Retarded Children. *Arkansas Journal for Health, Physical Education, and Recreation* 12:8–10, 1977.

Vodola, T. M. *Motor Disabilities or Limitations.* Oakhurst, NJ: Township of Ocean School District, 1976.

Wessel, J. A. *I CAN: Primary Skills.* Northbrook, IL: Hubbard, 1976.

Wessel, J. A., Project Director. *I CAN: Sport, Leisure and Recreation Skills.* Northbrook, IL: Hubbard, 1980.

CHAPTER 5

Test Selection and
Administration Insights

A valid and reliable assessment process takes into consideration three factors that influence student performance: (1) the demands of the task, (2) the unique history and characteristics that the student brings to the task, and (3) the factors inherent in the assessment process and setting. Assessment is not merely the administration of a test, it is a complex process of gathering information to help understand a student's motor behaviors in the *current ecology* (Salvia and Ysseldyke 1981). A major part of a comprehensive developmental/adapted physical education assessment process involves gathering information apart from formal testing procedures. Parents and teachers' observations of a student's movement behaviors are critical sources of assessment information. Assessment is a process of gathering, evaluating, interpreting, and appraising information about a student's motor performance.

Ways to Gather Information

Information about a child's motor performance can be gathered in a variety of ways relative to each student's unique situation. Regardless of the method used, we are measuring the student's attributes of motor performance and are *not* judging the student as a personality.

In educational settings, *formal tests* and *informal tests* are valuable tools for gathering information. In determining which assessment instrument or process to use, the purpose of the assessment should be considered. Whether the assessment is for (1) screening, (2) placement, (3) instructional planning, or (4) reviewing progress determines which formal and informal test procedures are most appropriate. The selection of formal and informal tests should be undertaken with extreme care to satisfy

41

the standards of validity and reliability described in Chapter 4. The methods selected to gather information should also be

1. Economical in terms of time and energy of student and tester
2. Appropriate to the student's unique characteristics, including physical, intellectual, and emotional development
3. Comprehensive in providing essential information to meet the purposes of the test (e.g., screening, placement, progress review)

Formal Tests

Frequently the terms test, measurement, and evaluation are used interchangeably. In this text, formal testing is considered to be the narrowest concept, meaning the presentation of a standard set of items that require a response. As a result of a student's movement responses to a given series of formal motor test items, we obtain a measure, that is, a numerical value, of a motor characteristic of that student.

In developmental/adapted physical education, the evaluator directs the student to execute a specific motor skill. The directions to the student must follow a standard procedure given in the administration guidelines of the test manual. When the student executes the desired motor skill, the evaluator assigns a score to the student's performance according to the test's standardized scoring procedure. An example of a formal test is a norm-referenced test, which we discuss in detail later in this chapter.

To ensure optimal validity and reliability, the evaluator must follow specifically the test's standardized procedures when administering formal tests. The evaluator should thoroughly study the test beforehand and learn the standardized procedures for giving test directions. When administering a formal motor skill test, the directions to the student are usually verbal and often involve demonstration. For some students who may have difficulty following directions, the evaluator may decide to rephrase the directions. Care should be taken when changing directions, and the evaluator should study the test manual guidelines regarding the presentation and possible alteration of verbal or visual directions.

In addition, formal tests usually have other standard procedures that must be followed in order to preserve standardized conditions. Besides administering the test, the tester must also establish the testing environment, introduce the student to the testing situation, use appropriate test equipment, and observe the student's motor performance according to the test's standardized procedures.

Test Environment

When establishing the test environment, use a simple checklist (Figure 5.1) to rate the adequacy of the testing room, space, and equipment. The appropriate test environment is crucial to administering a formal motor skill test. Many of the student's responses require space adequate for ball bouncing, throwing, running, jumping, or

Environment Checklist

Room	Test requirement	Optimal	Adequate	Poor
Ceiling height				
Distance				
Lighting				
Temperature/ventilation				
Noise level				
Freedom from distractions				
Breakable items				
Windows				
Floor surface				
Safety				
Unnecessary furniture				

Figure 5.1. Test environment checklist.

performing floor exercises. To promote awareness and support for the developmental/adapted physical education program, the evaluator should inform school administrators of any unique requirements for the test environment.

Preparing the Student

An important consideration in preparing to administer a formal test is introducing the student to the testing situation. Test scheduling, the physical needs of the student, and the student's psychological preparation are all vital considerations. The administration of a formal test is usually scheduled by the tester in cooperation with the classroom or physical education teacher. Whether the student will be missing a difficult subject or a favorite subject is a compromise decision between the teacher, the tester, and, when appropriate, the student.

Before beginning the test, considering the physical needs of the student is vital. Basic needs such as hunger, thirst, and a visit to the restroom should be met, so the student's attention is not distracted from the test situation by an unmet need. Shoelaces should be tied securely for optimal safety. If the student's handicapping condition requires an orthopedic, supportive, or other device, the tester must consider the option of testing with or without such devices. For example, should a student who wears leg braces remove them for the test? What about glasses, hearing aids, walkers, canes, or a communication board? Once again, the tester must consider the purpose of the assessment. If the purpose is to evaluate current motor skill functioning in a real-world situation, then devices should be kept in place to maximize validity.

Preparing the student psychologically for the test is also important. According to Anastasi (1976), establishing rapport with the student should arouse the student's interest in the test, elicit the student's cooperation, and ensure that he or she follows the standardized test directions. The tester will find it helpful to obtain some prior information about the student including the following:

1. Unique behavior problems that may interfere with the test
2. Special reinforcement methods that may help the student attend to the test
3. Particular topics that may motivate the student
4. Successful method of communicating directions

Such information can be of tremendous benefit to the tester in establishing a good working relationship with the student.

Upon initiating a formal test, the tester first introduces himself or herself to the student. The introduction should be friendly and communicate pleasure at the meeting. Second, the tester asks the student about himself or herself (e.g., What is your name? age? grade? favorite activities?) Focusing interest on the student should help the student relax and also provides the tester with some useful information about the student's style of communication (e.g., monosyllabic, voluble) and about the student's ability to participate in simple conversation. Third, the tester conveys the purpose of the test without raising unnecessary anxiety and states where in the school building she or he is taking the student. Telling the student that the purpose is "to do some work or exercises together in the gym" presents the setting as a work situation, rather than a play situation, which might be inferred if the tester said, "Today we're going to play some games in the gym." Students may not present a best effort if they believe that the testing situation is merely play. On the other hand, the term "test" should be used cautiously, since past experiences with failures may cause anxiety that could negatively influence the test results. Fourth, the tester should attempt to explain exactly what will happen during the test. Telling the student what is to come will help reduce the student's anxious feelings.

Formal tests usually include a set of instructions to be given at the start of test administration. Sometimes, because of the student's unique characteristics, the tester will have to devise a special set of instructions in a language appropriate to the age and ability level of the student. Pretest instructions should include information about the length of the test, the types of test activities, an indication of test difficulty, whether or not the tester will be able to help, and an indication of whether or not some tests will be timed. Fifth, the student should be encouraged to indicate any discomfort or to ask questions about anything not understood. Now is the time to make sure that the student understands the instructions and is not upset. The purpose of establishing a good rapport with the student is to create a pleasant, calm, unhurried atmosphere, which will encourage the student to put forth the best effort. It is also helpful during a formal test situation for the tester to encourage the student with comments such as "Good job," "You're doing nicely," or "That was a hard one." The tester should continue to observe carefully to determine when a student simply cannot perform a task and when anxiety, lack of confidence, or lapse in attention may be interfering with the test performance.

Administering a Formal Test

When administering a formal test, it is crucial to follow the test manual guidelines for administering and scoring. The formal, standardized conditions of the test will be violated if the tester departs from the guidelines. According to Salvia and Ysseldyke (1981, p. 35),

> The examiner must at all times administer tests exactly according to directions. Standardized tests were meant to be given in exactly the same way each time. Departure from standardized procedures destroys the meaning of test scores by rendering norms useless. Test users must not coach children on test items before administering the test; they must not alter time limits.

The tester should consult the test manual about rules for repeating directions or the questioning of responses, and should avoid the temptation to coach a student during a formal test. Although questioning and encouragement are permissible when administering formal tests, the tester must never coach the student. Coaching is considered helping or even teaching the desired response. It invalidates the student's response, because each test item was designed and normed on students who did not receive coaching.

Recording Responses

The manuals for formal tests include directions for recording student responses. Usually a formal test has a format or record form for recording. Once the form is completed, the test record is known as the *test protocol.* The test protocol is the original record of a student's responses during a formal test. Testers are advised to keep the protocol hidden from the student's view during the test, because seeing errors could affect the remaining students' performances. When administering a formal motor skills test, we suggest placing the record form on a clipboard with an opaque cover to conceal the responses. Motor skills tests require that the tester watch the student's performance and score the response simultaneously. Because accurately following the scoring guidelines is vital, the demand that the tester make on-the-spot decisions about the response requires special care in scoring both quickly and accurately. The tester should take the time to study the recording process thoroughly and know what to look for when watching a student performance. Most formal tests also provide a space on the form to record informal observations about the student's test behavior or to make comments about unique characteristics of the student's motor skill performance. This information can be useful in evaluating the success of the test situation and in further evaluating possible problems the student may have, such as orthopedic, vision, or hearing difficulties.

Informal Tests

In classrooms, physical education settings, playgrounds, and other natural settings, we use informal test procedures to gather information about a student's motor characteristics. In contrast to formal tests, informal test processes generally focus on a student's motor skill performance in relation to the demands of his or her environment. Informal assessments allow the tester to collect samples of movement behavior from the natural settings in which the child uses gross motor skills. Informal assessment procedures are important complements to formal tests. For some students with unique physical, emotional, intellectual, or sensory impairments, informal tests may constitute the only appropriate means of assessment. These tests usually yield information vital to making instructional decisions. They can also provide information for initial motor screening and assist in making placement decisions for developmental/adapted physical education programs.

Advantages and Disadvantages of Informal Tests

There is a wide variety of informal tests, including observation checklists, task analyses, informal inventories, rating scales, interviews, and questionnaires. Many informal tests are available commercially, or teachers may want to design their own, being careful to meet adequate standards of reliability and validity. One of the major advantages of informal assessment procedures is their relevance to teaching. Table 5.1 describes some different types of informal tests and their possible relation to the teaching setting.

Some disadvantages of informal tests are (1) they are often time-consuming to design and use, (2) information is usually not available concerning reliability or validity, and (3) they are not particularly useful in providing information about student performance in relation to performance of peers.

Selecting Informal Tests

There are several considerations when selecting an informal test for a developmental/adapted physical education program. First, the informal test must provide the needed information (i.e., screening, progress review, and so forth). Second, the tester should consider the relative efficiency of administering an informal test, including the time required for design and administration. Third, the most difficult and often the most important consideration is test quality. In contrast to formal test procedures that ensure a reasonable degree of technical accuracy in terms of reliability and validity, little information is usually available about the quality of informal motor tests. Most commercial informal motor skill tests are not standardized, and few contain validity and reliability information. When informal tests are designed by teachers, there can be no assurance about the quality of the procedures because the technical adequacy is not known.

When selecting informal tests, the two factors of quality that should be considered are content validity and reliability. The content validity of an informal test can be determined by examining the appropriateness of the motor test items for the content to be evaluated, the range of motor behavior included in the assessment, and the ways in which the items assess the motor skill content.

Reliability is another important quality factor when selecting informal motor tests. Many informal assessments of motor performance require someone to observe the student's movements and rate or score the student's motor performance. The tester must be relatively confident not only that his or her ratings of the student's performance are accurate, but also that another evaluator would obtain the same results if identical procedures were used with the student. We recommend that the tester estimate the interrater reliability of the informal motor test by calculating percent of agreement as described in Chapter 4.

Observation

Observation of a student's performance in a physical education class provides the most common basis for referral to developmental/adapted physical education programs. When, however, a classroom teacher notes a potential motor problem during casual class observation, employing more systematic observation methods may be appropriate. Informal observation allows the teacher to gather information about specific motor skill behaviors such as endurance, strength, locomotor patterns, agility,

Table 5.1. Informal Assessment Methods[a]

Informal Assessment Method	Description	Relation to Physical Education Instruction
Observation	Direct measure of student motor behavior	Determination of present levels of performance Documentation of student progress
Criterion-referenced tests	Direct measure of student performance on a specific motor task under specific conditions and with criteria for success	Determination of present levels of performance Documentation of student progress
Task analyses	Evaluation of a motor skill to locate motor subtasks appropriate for instruction	Direction for selection of appropriate criterion-referenced or informal tests Direction for selection of annual goals and objectives
Checklists, rating scales, and questionnaires	Evaluation of student performance based on accumulation of past experiences with student	Estimation of present levels of performance in physical education

[a]Adapted from J. McLoughlin and R. Lewis, *Assessing Special Students: Strategies and Procedures.* Columbus, OH: Charles E. Merrill, 1981.

eye-hand coordination, and social behaviors in group participation. Such observations are a source of vital information that often cannot be obtained from other assessment procedures. For example, a teacher may be concerned about the way a student continually "bumps" into other children during loosely structured large-group activities in the gymnasium. This behavior may be difficult to assess with a formal test, but informal observation methods help the teacher specify, record, and analyze the behavior as it occurs in the natural setting.

There are two different observation methods. The teacher's choice may depend on the desired outcome of the observation. The first method, *continuous recording* (Wallace and Larsen 1978) is used when a teacher chooses to observe all of the motor behaviors and related behaviors of a student during a specified time period. Figure 5.2 is an example of a continuous observation describing Dan's behavior during a 30-minute physical education class. Dan's teacher wanted Dan observed because of apparent clumsiness. In analyzing the results of the observation, Dan's clumsiness appears to stem from multiple intervening factors, including problems of listening and following directions, arm-shoulder strength, leg strength, eye-hand coordination, and attention-seeking behavior.

Continuous observations carried out by recording brief accounts of motor-related events during a specified time period can provide valuable information about the situational factors and the interactions involved in the student's behaviors. Continuous recording is time-consuming and difficult to execute since watching and writing are difficult to do simultaneously. Although it would be appropriate for the student's classroom teacher to conduct the observation, this is nearly impossible because it requires that the observer be freed from all other duties to focus full attention on the student.

For these reasons the second type of observation, *specific behavior observation*, may be more feasible and efficient. When specific motor behaviors are to be observed, the tester must be careful to describe those motor behaviors in observable and measurable terms. For example, a teacher may be interested in observing a student's physical strength and endurance during a physical education class. These physical fitness skills can best be documented if described in language such as: "Mary walks when others run," or "The ball Mary threw does not cross the center line." After the behavior has been specified, the tester must determine how it will be measured. Hammill and Bartel (1978) suggest several possible ways to measure specific observed behaviors. It may be of primary interest whether the behavior occurs at all. For example, the teacher may want to know whether or not Mary falls during physical education class. Data can also be collected on the number of times a behavior occurs. For example, the teacher may want to know the frequency of Mary's requests to "skip out" of a particular physical activity. Figure 5.3 demonstrates two methods of recording specific observational data: by recording events and by recording duration of a specified event.

Criterion-Referenced Tests and Task Analyses

Criterion-referenced tests (CRTs) are another form of informal assessment. They compare a student's motor performance to some criterion rather than to the perfor-

Student _Dan Brown_   Date _October 19, 1983_

Observer _Mr. Johnson_

Activity Observed _4th grade P.E. class, lesson on volleying with beachballs_

Reason for Observation _Teacher has reported that Dan seems clumsy, is inattentive and disruptive to class._

Time	Event
10:30–10:32	Dan comes into gym with group, wanders to equipment box while students sit in squads. Teacher tells Dan to sit in his squad.
10:32–10:35	Dan fidgets, wiggles, gazes around the gym as teacher gives directions for warm-ups.
10:35–10:38	Sit-ups: Dan pulls on his pant legs to sit up—does five this way.
10:38–10:40	Push-ups: Dan does not lift stomach from floor, but moves head up and down.
10:40–10:42	Jumping jacks: Arms O.K. but feet jump straight up and down without changing width.
10:42–10:45	Dan watches, then follows his squad as they move to their volleyball practice area. Dan is last to be assigned a partner.
10:45–10:49	Dan and partner begin "volleying" to each other—Dan either hits the ball too hard or misses the ball—spends extra time retrieving ball. Partner is frustrated.
10:49–10:52	Dan has wandered into another "squad's" practice area and interrupts the activity. Teacher leads Dan back to his partner.
10:52	Dan stops as teacher gives directions.
10:53–10:55	Dan follows squad members to their side of net (back row)—students begin volleying beachball. Dan watches, does not attempt to hit the ball when near.
10:55–10:57	Dan is in front row, and tries to volley, but hits ball with fist into the net; other times, Dan tries but misses.
10:57–11:00	Dan grabs ball as students begin to line up—kicks ball across gym. Teacher tells him to get ball; he retrieves it, then is last to line up.

Figure 5.2. Example of a continuous recording carried out during a 30-minute physical education class.

Method 1: Event Recording

Behavior:	John complains of being tired in physical education class.
Measurement:	Tally number of times (frequency) John verbally complains of being tired in physical education class.
When Measured:	Physical education class (9:30–10:00 a.m.) on 5 consecutive school days.

Day 1	Day 2	Day 3	Day 4	Day 5
~~HH~~ /	////	~~HH~~	///	~~HH~~

Total = 23 times in 5 class periods

Method 2: Duration Recording

Behavior:	Lori gazes away or walks away from physical activity.
Measurement:	How long (duration) Lori either looks away or walks away from the required physical activity.
When Measured:	During physical education class (9:30–10:00 a.m.) on 5 consecutive school days.

Day 1	Day 2	Day 3	Day 4	Day 5
9:30–9:35	9:30–9:37	9:32–9:36	9:30–9:36	9:30–9:34
9:42–9:48	9:40–9:43	9:42–9:47	9:41–9:49	9:40–9:44
9:50–9:56	9:49–9:54	9:48–9:52	9:53–9:58	9:48–9:52
		9:54–9:57		

| Total 17 min | 15 min | 16 min | 19 min | 12 min |

Total = 79 minutes in 5 class periods (150 minutes)

Figure 5.3. Two methods of specific behavior observation carried out by recording (method 1) number of times an event occurs during a given period and (method 2) duration of occurrences of a prespecified event during a given period.

mance of other students (as in formal norm-referenced tests). Criterion-referenced tests will be discussed fully later in this chapter.

Another method of informal motor skill assessment is task analysis. This technique can be used both for assessment of present level of performance and for instructional planning. Task analysis is defined by Howell et al. (1979, p. 81) as "the process of isolating, sequencing, and describing all the essential components of a task."

Conducting a task analysis involves a three-step process: (1) breaking down the motor behavior into essential subtasks, (2) arranging the subtasks in sequence, and (3) describing each subtask in the sequence as an instructional objective. Task analysis is valuable in planning and breaking down instruction into a sequence of teachable units. As an informal motor assessment technique, it can be used when motor skills are problematic for a student. The motor skill is analyzed in a sequence of subtasks (or submovements). The student's ability to perform each submovement is then assessed to discover at which steps of the sequence the student needs additional instruction, perhaps through a developmental/adapted physical education program. The *I CAN* program (Wessel 1976) is an example of a physical education program based on task analysis. Figure 5.4 presents examples from the *I CAN* program. Task analyses like those described can be used as a type of assessment. The submovements then become the objectives for which criterion-referenced tests are developed.

Other Informal Assessment Methods

Other types of informal motor tests include checklists, rating scales, interviews, and questionnaires. These assessment procedures incorporate techniques that allow access to otherwise unobservable behaviors. The teacher may be interested in gathering information about a student's attitudes and opinions or in obtaining information about the student's developmental history. Neither attribute can be observed directly.

Checklists.   Checklists provide a method of informal assessment in physical education settings. The tester quickly scans a descriptive list of motor behaviors and checks whether or not the behaviors apply to the student. Checklists can be used easily by teachers, parents, and even students. Developmental profiles are often in a checklist format. The assumption underlying the use of such lists is that the tester has carefully observed the student and is able by means of checking to describe the student's current or past behavior. Checklists are also an excellent format for gathering information not readily available in the physical education setting. They can be used to collect valuable information from parents about the child's developmental history, from physicians or therapists about medical concerns, or from parents or others about the child's motor performance in home and community settings. Information from former teachers and other professionals as well as current observations and records of progress can be gathered by means of checklists like those in Figure 5.5.

Rating Scales.   Another informal assessment tool is the use of rating scales. Rating scales enable the tester to express opinions and judgments. They allow the tester to evaluate or rate a student's motor performance, instead of merely reporting observations as with checklists. The assumption underlying the use of rating scales is that the tester has carefully observed the student and is able to form accurate, professional judgments. One common type of rating scale is a numerical scale based on the premise that 1 means low or poor performance, 3 means average or acceptable performance, and 5 means high or superior performance for the student's age. An example of a numerical rating scale of motor skills is presented in Figure 5.6. Rating

I CAN

PERFORMANCE OBJECTIVE:
TO DEMONSTRATE A FUNCTIONAL LEVEL OF STAMINA AND HEART/LUNG STRENGTH AND ENDURANCE

SKILL LEVELS	FOCAL POINTS FOR ACTIVITY
1. To perform an endurance walk/jog with assistance.	Given a verbal request, a demonstration and physical assistance (stand beside student, grasp hand or arm), the student can jog and/or walk on a clearly marked endurance jogging course for the age-appropriate time period (see Table 3) without assistance.
2. To perform an endurance walk/jog without assistance.	Given a verbal request, a demonstration, and a clearly marked course, the student can jog and/or walk an endurance jogging course for the age-appropriate time period (see Table 3) without assistance.
3. To perform an endurance jog without assistance.	Given a verbal request, a demonstration, and a clearly marked course, the student can jog for the age-appropriate time period (see Table 3) without assistance.
4. To demonstrate an appropriate level of stamina and heart/lung endurance.	Given a verbal request, a demonstration, and a command to "start" and "stop," the student can demonstrate an appropriate level of stamina in the following manner: a. Beginning and stopping after the required time b. Meeting the minimal performance criteria for individual's age and sex. (See Physical Fitness Performance Criteria, Table 3.)
5. To maintain an appropriate level of stamina and heart/lung endurance.	Given the ability to perform the endurance jog at the appropriate age and sex criteria (see Table 3), the student can maintain that criteria (or achieve the new criteria in instances where a new age category is achieved) over a 12-week period.

Figure 5.4. Example of task analysis from the *I CAN* program. From *I CAN Primary Skills*, Janet A. Wessel, Director. Reprinted with permission of the publisher, HUBBARD.

Sample 1: Fundamental Motor Skills
a. Locomotor Skills
   Walking
   ___1. even gait
   ___2. heel-toe
   ___3. arm opposition
   ___4. erect posture
   Running
   ___1. smooth pattern
   ___2. heel-toe
   ___3. arm opposition
   ___4. knee bend 90 degrees
   ___5. narrow support base
   Broad Jump
   ___1. prepare with forward bend, knees bent
   ___2. prepare with arms swinging way back
   ___3. arms swing forward and up during jump
   ___4. lands feet first, assumes standing position

Sample 2: Motor Development Inventory
Static Balance*
___Stands momentarily
___Stands alone
___Stands alone well
   Stands on one foot with help:
___   Right
___   Left
___Squats in play
___Balances on one foot, 1 sec
___Stands on tiptoe demonstrated
___Balances on one foot, 5 sec, 2 or 3 trials
___Balances on one foot, 10 sec, 2 or 3 trials
___Balances on tiptoes, 10 sec with hands on hips, 2 or 3 trials

---

Sample 3: Physical Education Referral Checklist
Directions: Read through the following list carefully and circle the number in front of each statement that describes a problem that the student displays during physical education class.
1 Easily distracted
2 Difficulty following directions
3 Body constantly moving
4 Loses balance easily
5 Locomotor patterns are jerky, awkward
6 Difficulty doing jumping tasks, shows poor gross body coordination
7 Is withdrawn
8 Drops the ball frequently
9 Frequently "bumps" into walls, other people
10 Low endurance, tires easily
11 Poor upper body strength
12 Often has physical complaints
13 Is noisy, disruptive
14 Difficulty following game strategies
15 Avoids or disrupts cooperative games
16 Seems disoriented

---

*M. Cohen and P. J. Gross, *The Developmental Resources*: Behavioral Sequences for Assessment and Program Planning, vol I. New York: Grune and Stratton, 1979, p. 140.

Figure 5.5. Sample motor behavior checklists.

Numerical Rating Scale
Fundamental Motor Skills (Locomotor)
   1—Poorly executed motor pattern (awkward, clumsy, off-balance)
   2—Basic motor pattern with inconsistency and some difficulty
   3—Average motor pattern for age level
   4—Smoothly integrated motor pattern
   5—Superior motor pattern with optimum speed, distance, accuracy
Directions: Circle the number that best describes the student's motor behavior.

1.	Walking	1	2	3	4	5
2.	Running	1	2	3	4	5
3.	Hopping	1	2	3	4	5
4.	Jumping (vertical)	1	2	3	4	5
5.	Jumping (horizontal)	1	2	3	4	5

Figure 5.6. Example of a numerical rating scale for evaluation of motor skills.

scales are sometimes useful in assessing student attitudes. Pupil progress can also be recorded on a rating scale with the teacher rating the student's motor performance as (a) improvement shown, (b) improvement needed, and so forth. This type of rating scale is used frequently on report cards.

Interviews and questionnaires.   These are two other methods of informal assessment. Designed to gather information about opinions, attitudes, and sometimes to amass facts, interviews are conducted orally while questionnaires are primarily written instruments. There is wide variety in the types of interviews and questionnaires, from the highly structured to those open-ended and flexible enough to allow for further exploration of relevant topics. Interviews and questionnaires can be designed to tap several different physical education domains and may be designed for students with varying levels of ability. Like other informal assessment procedures, interviews and questionnaires have as an underlying assumption that the tester has accurately gathered and recorded the information and will report the information correctly. Questionnaires are useful in gathering information from parents about the child's medical history, birth history, infant development and other developmental history. Interviews and questionnaires can also be used to gather information directly from students. For example, a series of questions could be designed to probe student opinions about their own physical education performance. Questions might include the following:

1.   Do you like physical education class? Why or why not?
2.   What activities in physical education do you like best?
3.   Which physical education activities do you like least?
4.   Which physical education activities are hardest for you?
5.   Do you participate in any physical activities outside of school? If so, what are they?

6. If you could change physical education today, what changes would you make?
7. Would you like special help with physical education?

The informal assessment tools, including checklists, rating scales, and question-naires, do not directly measure student motor behavior, but are instead dependent on information gathered from the informants. The value of that information hinges on the accuracy of the motor information provided by the informant. Problems in using informal measures include faulty memory of past events, inadequate obser-vation of current events, and faulty judgments. Informal assessment of motor skills is most valuable in its relevance to physical education instruction. Because teachers develop and design their own informal assessment questions, immediate results are available to help make instructional decisions.

Interpreting Informal Tests

Interpretation of informal test results is often difficult, especially when the quality of the informal procedure is relatively unknown. Any criterion established for inter-preting informal results is selected judgmentally, and that makes translation into meaningful instruction difficult. Furthermore, most informal tests sample only a few skills in the entire physical education domain, making it difficult to use informal tests as a basis for establishing valid directions for programming developmental/adapted physical education. Even with these limitations, informal assessment is a necessary and valuable component of the comprehensive developmental/adapted physical ed-ucation program. The teacher should remember, however, that results of informal assessment procedures must be interpreted with caution and with consideration for the specific student's unique strengths and needs.

Informal assessment is a valuable complement to formal, standardized tests. For example, if standardized motor test results reveal that a student's motor ability is below average range for her or his age level, then informal assessment procedures such as criterion-referenced tests and checklists can provide vital information about the specific motor skills the student has acquired and those skills for which special instruction is needed. In this way, informal motor tests can assist in the total motor assessment process.

Norm-Referenced and Criterion-Referenced Tests

Norm-referenced and criterion-referenced tests are not the only types of tests that a teacher can select. Such a dichotomous approach to motor assessment would nar-row unnecessarily our perspective, since a great variety of approaches to motor as-sessment exist. One characteristic that norm-referenced and criterion-referenced tests have in common is that they are both objective. Each is characterized by a standard set of answers and scoring procedures. Objective tests do not permit attitudes, opin-ions, or idiosyncrasies of the tester to affect scoring. Since norm-referencing and cri-terion-referencing represent a major portion of assessment procedures, we will dis-cuss the advantages and disadvantages of each.

Norm-Referenced Tests

Tests that examine a student's motor performance in relation to the motor performance of a representative group are *norm-referenced tests*. Norm-referenced tests are frequently confused with "formal tests" and "standardized tests." As discussed in the previous section, norm-referenced tests are a kind of formal test. A standardized test is one in which all students are given the same tasks under uniform directions. In norm-referenced tests, "norm" refers to the test performance of a sample of subjects with characteristics similar to those subjects for whom the test was designed (for example, eight-year-old girls of mixed races from a range of economic backgrounds and from all geographic areas of the U.S.).

A norm-referenced motor test is used when a teacher wants to administer a test that predicts with great accuracy the students who have high, average, and low motor proficiency. If a teacher wants to determine the relative position (high or low) of a student's motor skill performance in relation to other students with similar characteristics, the teacher should select a well-constructed norm-referenced motor test as the appropriate instrument. Norm-referenced tests can be useful tools for guiding placement decisions in developmental/adapted physical education programs, for the purposes of screening, and for program evaluation.

Test Construction

A norm-referenced motor test is designed to determine an individual's rank-order position in relation to the motor performance of a norm group (peers) who have also taken the test. To be an accurate assessment of an individual's relative position, a wide range of motor performances must be included. A norm-referenced motor test is constructed around the author's choice of components from the motor domain. The AAHPERD Youth Fitness Test, for example, contains items designed to test physical fitness, while the Bruininks-Oseretsky Test was developed to assess overall motor proficiency. Norm-referenced tests are usually developed to assess general areas of motor performance, rather than specific physical education skill content.

The test author's challenge is to develop clear, reliable, and valid test items representing the particular attributes of motor performance to be assessed. Once the motor test items are developed, they must then be piloted on a sample of subjects representative of those for whom the test is being designed. When the data from the sample have been collected, it is analyzed item by item to determine which items to retain. The best items are judged to be those that produce the greatest diversity of scores. Items that were responded to either correctly or incorrectly by too many subjects are usually eliminated. Popham (1978) notes that the test items on which students perform best are likely to be the tasks that have received the greatest emphasis during physical education instruction. The resulting norm-referenced tests, therefore, tend *not* to include tasks that measure the major physical education emphases of schools.

Following this procedure, the revised motor test is administered to a group of students representative of those for whom the test was designed (norm group). Lastly, studies of reliability and validity are conducted on the final version of the test.

Statistics of Norm-Referenced Tests

A norm-referenced test is based on the assumption that the motor behaviors we are interested in measuring are normally distributed. Three measures of *central tendency* describe the sample distribution of test scores: the mean, the mode, and the median. These three terms refer to typical, or average, performance. Teachers who wish to examine generally how well a group of students performed will use the *mode*, which is the most frequently occurring score. To determine the midpoint of a distribution, a teacher calculates the *median*, the point at which half of the scores are higher and half are lower. The median is helpful in describing distributions that contain unusually high or low scores. Most often the *mean* is used to describe the central tendency of a distribution. The mean is actually the arithmetic average of a distribution, obtained by summing the scores and dividing the sum by the number of scores. When using measures of central tendency, remember that these terms are appropriate for describing a group but are not necessarily useful in describing an individual group member.

Measures of *variability* describe how much the scores in a distribution vary from one another. The most common description of variability in an educational setting is the *standard deviation*, a calculation based on the degree to which the scores deviate from the mean. We refer to a score as being a certain number of standard deviations above (+) or greater than the mean, or a certain number below (−) or less than the mean. In normal distributions, a precise relationship exists between the standard deviation and the percentage of students whose scores fall within one standard deviation above or below the mean (Figure 5.7). For any normal distribution, 68.2% of the student scores will be between +1 standard deviation and −1 standard deviation.

Standard deviations can be useful in determining cutoff points for placement in a developmental/adapted physical education program. A school district may decide, for example, that a score of two standard deviations below the mean on a norm-referenced motor skills test along with other vital assessment information meets the criteria for eligibility in a developmental/adapted physical education program.

Norm-Referenced Test Scores

The number of correct responses on a motor test constitutes the *raw scores* that are basic to calculating descriptive data. In norm-referenced tests, raw scores take on meaning when they are compared with the scores of students in the norm group. The result of this comparison is a type of score called a *norm*, which is a description of the performance of that specific group. When discussing norm-referenced test scores, the normal curve, as shown in Figure 5.7, is used to illustrate the relationship of the types of scores to one another and to the curve.

Percentile Norms. Percentile norms are used frequently when reporting educational diagnostic data. A percentile norm tells the percentage of a norm group that falls at or below a specific score. If a student received a raw score of 20, which the test norms indicate is better than 45 percent of the norm group, then the student's percentile rank is 45.

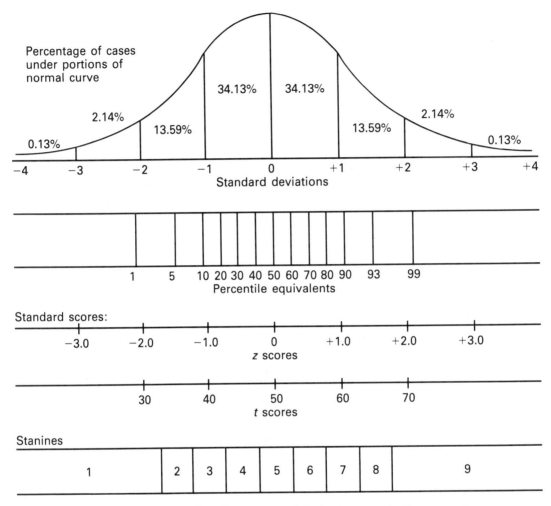

Figure 5.7. Relationship of various types of derived scores to the normal curve.

One of the advantages of using percentiles is that they are relatively easy to understand. Lay persons unfamiliar with testing procedures can readily understand that a percentile of 45 means that a child demonstrated near-average motor performance as compared with the norm group. Another advantage of using percentile norms is that the norm reference group has characteristics similar to those of the student taking the test. On the AAHPERD Youth Fitness Test, for example, the score of a 12-year-old girl is based on a comparison with the 12-year-old girls in the norm group. For each age group for which the test is designed, a set of percentile norms should be available. A third advantage of percentile scores is that they can be easily used to compare a student's performance in several subtest areas or across various subject areas. Percentile scores on a motor ability test, for example, can be examined with percentile scores in reading and mathematics achievement. A student who is at the 10th percentile in motor ability, the 60th percentile in reading, and the 45th in mathematics, demonstrates relatively low motor performance compared with other subject areas.

One caution should be noted, however, when using percentile scores: a percentile norm does not have equal units at all points on the scale. For example, percentiles of 48 on speed and agility and 53 on balance represent very similar raw scores. In contrast, the same 5-point difference at the 2nd and 7th percentiles represents correspondingly large differences. A distribution that closely approximates normality should reveal a clustering of percentile scores toward the middle of the distribution, as is evident in Figure 5.7.

Standard Scores.   Standard score norms describe the distance of a student's test score from the mean in terms of standard deviations. Examples of standard scores are *t* scores and *z* scores, illustrated in Figure 5.7. Another standard score that is used more frequently in educational settings is the *stanine* score. As indicated in Figure 5.7, stanine scores have a mean of 5 and a standard deviation of approximately 2. Like percentile scores, standard scores carry uniform size characteristics from test to test. Standard scores should be used with caution, however, because in some tests the scores are contaminated by other variables, such as grade-basing rather than age-basing.

Developmental Norms.   Developmental norms, or age-score norms, are used frequently in motor assessment methods. These test scores are meaningful because they indicate how far along the normal motor developmental continuum a student has progressed. Developmental norms can provide information such as whether a 6-year-old boy's current motor behavior is approximately like that of other 6-year-old boys. Developmental information is being increasingly emphasized in assessment in developmental/adapted physical education programs. Determining where in the development of a motor skill a student's current performance is, as compared with age peers, provides vital information in guiding the development of individualized education programs. Because developmental scores do not carry uniform meaning from test to test and are not of uniform size, their usefulness is somewhat limited for purposes of comparison in the educational setting.

Criterion-Referenced Tests

These tests have become increasingly popular in recent educational and behavioral psychology practices. While norm-referenced tests indicate a student's relative status in motor skill development in comparison with a peer sample, criterion-referenced motor tests measure a student's motor skill development in terms of absolute levels of mastery. Criterion-referenced tests compare a student's motor performance to some predetermined criterion, rather than to the performance of other students. These tests are usually curriculum based, to determine which physical education skills a student has mastered. Criterion-referenced tests simply measure the aspects of motor behavior that a student can and cannot do. The tests do not provide information about whether the student's motor performance is average for his or her age.

Test Construction

Criterion-referenced tests are relatively easy to construct, can be used to measure any motor behavior, and are directly relevant to physical education instruction. Specific instructional questions are used to generate criterion-referenced tests. For example, a physical education teacher may want to know whether John can dribble a ball ten times consecutively, whether he can demonstrate accuracy in a volleyball serve, or whether he can complete 25 bent-knee curl-ups. Any of these physical education questions can be answered by constructing a criterion-referenced physical education test. Howell, Kaplan, and O'Connell (1979, pp. 96–97) suggest the following guidelines for developing criterion-referenced tests:

1. Decide what specific questions you want answered about a student's motor skill behavior. What motor skills do you want to test?
2. Write a performance objective that describes how you are going to test the student. It should include (a) what motor behavior the student must do, (b) under what conditions the student will engage in this motor skill, and (c) how well the student must perform in order to pass the test.
3. Use the performance objective to help you write your criterion-referenced test. All of the necessary test components are present in your objective. These components are (a) the directions for administration and scoring, (b) the criterion for passing the test, and (c) the materials, equipment, and necessary setting.

Questions about the student's motor behavior form the basis for developing a criterion-referenced test. These questions may be generated from (1) performance in general motor areas on a norm-referenced test, (2) analysis and observation of a student's performance during physical education class, or (3) class records of progress in a physical education curriculum.

Once the questions are formulated in specific terms, they are used to write performance objectives. According to Mager (1975), performance objectives should include

1. Desired motor behavior stated in observable terms
2. Conditions under which the motor behavior should occur
3. Criterion for acceptable motor performance

For example, a physical education teacher may be interested in determining if a student can "kick a ball." This is an important question, but it needs to be further defined. "Kicking a ball" can be interpreted as a toe-kick, a kick for distance, a kick for accuracy, or a soccer dribble. The question should be specifically stated to describe the skill the teacher is interested in, such as: The student, when requested by the teacher to "kick the ball," will kick a 10-inch ball into a 6-foot-wide, 3-foot-high goal area, using a shoelace kick, from a distance of 12 ft, four out of five times.

The criterion in this objective is "four out of five times." The criterion can be determined by identifying same-aged students whom you feel possess the skill desired and measuring their performance against the objective. The minimum level of performance by these students then becomes the standard for passing that item on a criterion-referenced test.

Figure 5.4 presented an example of a performance objective from Wessel's *I CAN* (1976) program. Each objective is tested by means of a criterion-referenced assessment as shown on the score sheet in Figure 5.8. If a student passes a criterion-referenced item, the teacher can assume that the student has mastered the performance objective assessed by the test. Physical education instruction may then progress to the next objective in the curriculum sequence. When a student does not pass a criterion-referenced item, testing should continue until the student passes an objective (usually lower in the sequence) to determine the next objective for instruction.

Teachers may design their own criterion-referenced tests to fit their instructional program, or they may use a commercially prepared test such as the *I CAN* program. Dunn's (1980) Data-Based Physical Education Curriculum and components of Project A.C.T.I.V.E. (Vodola 1974) also contain criterion-referenced motor tests. These tests, since they are objective-based, are useful in writing individualized education programs.

Statistics From Criterion-Referenced Tests

The quality of criterion-referenced tests is generally unknown and difficult to measure. Because of their highly skill-specific nature and predominately local usage, few data are available on standardization, reliability, or validity. The *I CAN* program has been nationally validated and studies of reliability have been conducted. A further attempt to standardize criterion-referenced physical education test items has been undertaken by Ulrich (1981). Examples of Ulrich's criterion-referenced test are included in Figure 5.9. Efforts such as Ulrich's are supported by Popham (1978, p. 171) who suggested: "Without comparative data, criterion-referenced measures will never win acceptance of the many citizens, legislators, and educators who are properly asking, 'Is the schools' performance good enough?'"

Criterion-Referenced Test Scores

Scores derived from criterion-referenced tests are directly interpretable in terms of the motor tasks on the test. Because criterion-referenced tests contain "standards," the scale common to these tests is the percentage of items correct. The administration and scoring of criterion-referenced tests should be explicit and objective to the extent that independent testers would obtain essentially the same scores for the same students (Ebel 1962). Criterion-referenced test scores specify the percentage of items in

Figure 5.8. *I CAN* class performance score sheet. From *I CAN Primary Skills*, Janet A. Wessel, Director. Reprinted with permission of the publisher, HUBBARD.

Equipment: A minimum of 30 feet of clear space, colored tape or other marking device Objective: Slide	Body turned sideways to desired direction					
	A step sideways followed by a slide of the trailing foot next to the lead foot					
		A short period where both feet are off the ground				
			Able to slide to the right and left side			
				Directions: Mark off a straight line. Ask student to do a slide 3 times to each side, staying on the line.		
Name	1	2	3	4	Comments	

Figure 5.9. An example of criterion-referenced assessment by Dale Ulrich, 1983.

a domain that the student can perform and are essentially raw scores. The raw scores obtained from criterion-referenced tests are meaningful if the motor content and the test specification are described as clearly and precisely as possible. In criterion-referenced tests, no derived scores are calculated because normative comparisons are not made.

Although the reliability of criterion-referenced tests may not be specified, Salvia and Ysseldyke (1981) stress the importance of examining the reliability of these tests. The tester should check the percentage of agreement among ratings, as described in Chapter 4.

Judging Technical Adequacy

Faced with a heterogeneous group of students to evaluate, and armed with a "mixed bag" of available motor tests, the physical educator may find test selection a frustrating dilemma. Not only are physical education teachers required to individualize instruction for nonhandicapped and handicapped students, but test selection requires teachers to be skilled in judging the technical adequacy of motor tests. For the physical educator who wants thorough assistance in evaluating tests, the following publications provide critical reviews: *Standards for Educational and Psychological Tests and Manuals* (APA Standards), Davis (1974), *The Eighth Annual Mental Measurements Yearbook,* Buros (1978), and *Assessment in Special and Remedial Education,* Salvia and Ysseldyke (1981). All provide valuable guidelines for judging the excellence of tests. A limitation of these resources, however, is that they focus primarily on psychological and academic tests, and provide only scant reviews of tests in the psychomotor domain. Although such resources have limitations, the test user's challenge is to be as critical and precise as possible when administering tests, understanding and interpreting results, and making decisions based on test results. Test users should review their skills according to the following qualifications adapted from Davis (1974):

1. Test users should have a general knowledge of measurement principles and the limitations of test interpretations.
2. Users should know their own qualifications and how well they match the qualifications required for the use of specific tests.
3. Users of psychomotor tests who are responsible for education decision making about students should have an understanding of psychomotor measurement and its validation.
4. Physical education program administrators are responsible for ensuring that all physical education teachers who are required to conduct assessments have received training appropriate to those responsibilities.
5. Anyone administering a test of motor skill development for decision-making purposes should be competent to administer the test. If unqualified, necessary training should be sought regardless of previous educational training.
6. Test users should seek to avoid biased or discriminatory practices in test selection, administration, and interpretation (especially bias of age, sex, cultural background, or handicapping condition).

Tests in general have received widely publicized criticism from both the professional and lay communities. Particular tests that are currently used in education have been criticized for their technical inadequacies (Bersoff 1973, Ebel 1974, Anastasi 1976, Salvia and Ysseldyke 1981). Some of these criticisms were summarized by Swanson and Watson (1982).

1. Technical inadequacy
2. Improper administration and interpretation
3. Impracticality for instructional purposes

4. Used for the wrong purposes
5. Racial and ethnic biases
6. Misconceptions of genetic endowment and learning ability
7. Invasion of privacy

Tests can be criticized as being technically inadequate when they fail to meet standards of reliability, validity, and normative characteristics. When selecting a motor test to provide information for instructional decision-making, the test user should check the test to examine whether it does the following:

1. Measures what it purports to measure
2. Obtains consistent, reliable information with minimal measurement error
3. Provides normative information about the characteristics of the population (e.g., age, grade, socioeconomic status)

The standards for validity and reliability discussed in Chapter 4 provide the basis for judgment of technical adequacy. Test authors are responsible for presenting evidence that the test has appropriate item content, is an acceptable measure of the motor skill components that it purports to measure, and has useful predictive validity in practical situations common to the test user's situation. In addition, the test manual should provide evidence of the consistency of test scores obtained by members of the test's standardization sample. The test user should examine the manual for data that indicates the test's relative freedom from measurement error and the average variation that can be expected in a particular student's score. The test manual should contain enough information to assure the user that test results cannot be attributed to departures from the standardized procedures for administration and scoring.

After examining the manual, the prospective user may have reason to be skeptical of a test's technical adequacy. Salvia and Ysseldyke (1981, p. 347) are critical in their review of perceptual-motor tests:

> What the majority of the research *has* shown is that most perceptual-motor tests are unreliable. We do not know what they measure, because they do not measure anything consistently. Unlike the majority of intelligence and achievement tests, the tests used to assess perceptual-motor skills in children are technically inadequate. And for the most part they are neither theoretically nor psychometrically sound. For example, they are designed to assess perceptual-motor abilities under the assumption that such abilities cause academic success or academic failure (see Salvia and Ysseldyke 1974). Or they are designed to assess hypothetical constructs like figure-ground perception and body image and differentiation but do not do so with consistency (see Salvia and Ysseldyke 1974). Or they may be based on criterion keying, an approach that can lead to logical fallacies of undistributed middle terms (all canaries eat birdseed; Esmeralda eats birdseed; therefore, Esmeralda is a canary).
>
> In short, the devices currently used to assess children's perceptual-motor skills are extremely inadequate. The real danger is that reliance on such tests in planning interventions for children may actually lead to assigning children to activities that do them absolutely no good.

Swanson and Watson (1982, p. 265) tend to agree with such criticisms of perceptual-motor tests:

> The results indicate, as have most test authors, that these instruments generally do not meet rigorous standards of reliability and validity and hence cannot be considered to be definitive diagnostic measures. This does not mean that they are not useful for clinical purposes and research as demonstrated by the profiles of learning-disabled readers.

While we agree that there is reason for concern about the technical adequacy of many psychomotor tests, we believe that existing tests can be helpful in light of the following considerations:

1. Criticisms of psychomotor tests are based on reviews of *perceptual-motor tests.* Other tests in the physical education field have not been included in such reviews, and many of these are technically adequate.
2. Test users should be sure that test selection is based on *clearly formulated objectives.* For example, if the objective is to test physical education skills of a 14-year-old student, the test user should ask: Will a perceptual-motor test fulfill that objective? Which assessment procedures would best provide the information I seek?
3. A score on any test should be interpreted as an *estimate* of motor skill performance under a given set of circumstances. Test scores should not be interpreted as some measure of an absolute motor characteristic, or as something permanent and generalizable to all other circumstances.
4. Test users must consider *more than one motor factor* for assessment, and the assessment of any given motor factor by *more than one method.*

When it appears that a test does not meet the standards of technical adequacy, the test user can take several courses of action. If a test is inadequate in validity, reliability, and standardization, it probably should not be used. The test may, however, contain specific items that are useful if administered individually. If, for example, you believe that a particular item testing balance would be helpful, the item can be administered if precautions are followed. First, check validity to see if the item does indeed test what you want it to test (e.g., dynamic balance). Second, determine interrater reliability for the item by calculating percentage of agreement. The item can be administered and scored by other testers or on different occasions to check reliability. Third, do not report the results of a single item comparatively if the standardization sample is inadequate. These guidelines can also be used for tests that are inadequate in one of the areas of validity, reliability, or standardization. If a test is reliable and valid but has an inadequate standardization sample for a given student, then comparison results should not be computed. The test user should examine instead the differences between the characteristics of the student to be tested and the characteristics of the individuals on whom the test norms were developed. The tester's responsibility is to decide whether the differences are so great that the test should not be used for that student. Salvia and Ysseldyke (1981, p. 366) provide a summary

of a review of the Purdue Perceptual-Motor Survey, which demonstrates the usefulness of such reviews:

> The Purdue Perceptual-Motor Survey is designed to provide qualitative information
> regarding the extent to which children demonstrate adequately developed perceptual-
> motor skills. Because standardization was limited, the survey cannot be used for the
> purpose of making normative comparisons. Although good test-retest reliability has
> been demonstrated, validity of the scale is questionable. Individual teachers must judge
> whether they are willing to accept the authors' contention that the development of
> adequate perceptual-motor skills is a necessary prerequisite to the acquisition of aca-
> demic skills. Such a claim is, to date, without support.

While the items were designed to test correlates of academic functioning, the Purdue
survey may have some valid motor items that could be used judiciously.

The guidelines we have suggested should be followed when selecting, administering, or interpreting tests and when transmitting such interpretations to others. It
is vital to remember that scores on motor tests must never be interpreted as representing innate, fixed abilities and characteristics of the student being tested. Also
important is the recognition that measurement error exists in any test score and must
be taken into account in test interpretations. Lastly, be sure to provide test interpretations that are based on technically adequate scores, are clear, and readily understandable by other members of the child-study team.

When No Appropriate Tests Are Available

Because of the wide variation among students who need motor assessment, no
single test can be adequate for all students. Not surprisingly, the test user will not
always find a single test that seems appropriate for a particular student. The evaluator
still has the responsibility, however, of conducting an appropriately comprehensive
physical education assessment that provides meaningful information for decision
making.

Figure 5.10 presents a systematic checklist for developing an appropriate assessment battery. The first step in conducting this assessment is to establish clearly defined motor domain objectives that fulfill the purpose of the assessment. Next, the
characteristics of the individual student are taken into consideration. Relevant cognitive, affective, and physical characteristics that affect the assessment should be considered. The results of the checklist can lead to the selection of an individualized
assessment battery. Figure 5.10 shows the results of completing the checklist for a
third grader with cerebral palsy.

The complex, individualized nature of physical education assessment of children
with handicaps is evident in this example. Assessment is a multifaceted process that
may or may not include commercially available tests, and when formal tests are not
available, informal measures become the vital instruments for information gathering.

Checklist Information	Types of Assessment
1. Purpose of Assessment? Instructional planning	Criterion-referenced tests, informal tests
2. Components of physical education? Fundamental motor skills Physical fitness Participation	Rating scales based on observation Baseline endurance rate, and physical therapist's evaluation of range of motion Observation of social integration, amount of movement, general attitude toward P.E.
3. Student Characteristics? Normal intellectually Shy, self-conscious Cerebral palsy, lower extremity, hip, knee, ankle spasticity. Wears short leg braces and uses quadruped canes.	Assessment should provide success and reinforcement Use normal task analyses for upper extremities, except where balance may interfere Parent interview Reports of physician, physical therapist Interview classroom teacher Observe P.E. classes, playground Most important is determination of level of play, participation, and amount of physical activity in natural environments

Figure 5.10. Checklist results used to determine an assessment battery.

References

Anastasi, A. *Psychological Testing*. New York: Macmillan, 1976.

Bersoff, D. Silk Purses into Sows' Ears: the Decline of Psychological Testing and a Suggestion for Its Redemption. *American Psychologist* 10: 892–899, 1973.

Buros, O. K., ed. *The Sixth Mental Measurements Yearbook*. Highland Park, NJ: Gryphon Press, 1965.

Buros, O. K., ed. *The Eighth Annual Mental Measurements Yearbook (Vols. 1 and 2)*. Highland Park, NJ: Gryphon Press, 1978.

Cohen, J. A., and Gross, P. J. *The Developmental Resource*, Vol. I. New York: Grune and Stratton, 1979.

Davis, F. *Standards for Educational and Psychological Tests and Manuals*. Washington, DC: American Psychological Association, 1974.

Dunn, J. M. et al., *A Data-based Gymnasium: A Systematic Approach to Physical Education for the Handicapped*. Instructional Development Corporation, Monmouth, OR, 1980.

Ebel, R. Content Standard Test Scores. *Educational and Psychological Measurement* 22: 15–25, 1962.

Ebel, R. Educational Tests: Valid? Biased? Useful? *Phi Delta Kappan* 57:83–88, 1974.

Hammill, D. D., and Bartel, N. R. *Teaching Children with Learning and Behavior Problems. (2nd ed.)*. Boston: Allyn and Bacon, 1978.

Howell, K., Kaplan, J., and O'Connell, C. *Evaluating Exceptional Children.* Columbus, OH: Charles E. Merrill, 1979.

Mager, R. F. *Preparing Instructional Objectives.* (2nd ed.) Belmont, CA: Fearon, 1975.

McLoughlin, J. A., and Lewis, R. B. *Assessing Special Students.* Columbus, OH: Charles E. Merrill, 1981.

Popham, W. J. *Criterion-Referenced Measurement.* Englewood Cliffs, NJ: Prentice-Hall, 1978.

Salvia, J., and Ysseldyke, J. *Assessment in Special and Remedial Education.* Boston: Houghton-Mifflin, 1981.

Swanson, H. L., and Watson, B. L. *Educational and Psychological Assessment of Exceptional Children.* St. Louis, MO: C. V. Mosby, 1982.

Vodola, T. M., Project Director. *All Children Totally Involved Exercising.* Oakhurst, NJ: Township of Ocean School District, 1974.

Wallace, G., and Larsen, S. *Educational Assessment of Learning Problems: Testing for Teaching.* Boston: Allyn and Bacon, 1978.

Wessel, J. A., Project Director. *I CAN: Primary Skills.* Northbrook, IL: Hubbard, 1976.

CHAPTER 6

Psychomotor Tests

The physical educator faced with the challenge of assessment can select from several types of tests. The evaluator will want to keep in mind that tests should be selected only when (1) they match the objectives and purpose of the assessment, (2) they test the motor characteristics that they are intended to measure, (3) they are reliable, consistent measures of motor performance, and (4) they are designed and standardized on a population similar to the student you are about to assess.

Developmental Tests

Developmental tests are norm-referenced standardized tests designed to evaluate how far along the normal motor developmental continuum a student has progressed. The use of developmental norms assumes that comparing the performance of a handicapped student to normal development is appropriate. This assumption must be considered carefully, and its validity questioned in cases of subjects with physical disabilities, severe or profound handicaps, or adult subjects with handicaps. Developmental scores, including age and grade equivalents, compare a student's performance across age or grade peer groups. Developmental norms are useful in clinical case studies, in initial motor development screening, and in longitudinal research of motor development. Cratty (1980, p. 77) advocates the use of a developmental approach in adapted physical education programs. Such an approach assumes that:

1. All children and youth go through roughly the same series of developmental tasks; the differences lie in the time of life during which the tasks may be encountered and mastered.

2.   To aid developmentally delayed children or youth, one should identify where (on one or more levels) the individual presently functions and should then attempt to take the individual further by presenting tasks that are developmentally just ahead of the present levels.

Cratty's advocacy of a developmental approach supports such long-standing proponents of the importance of studying motor development as Rarick, Roberton, Seefeldt, and Haubenstricker whose views are described in Kelso and Clark's *The Development of Movement Control and Co-ordination* (1982).

Some frequently used standardized development tests include the Denver Developmental Screening Test, the Lincoln-Oseretsky Motor Development Scale, the Bayley Scales of Infant Development, and the Gesell Developmental Schedules. In this section we will briefly review three standardized development tests and how they can be used in adapted physical education programs.

Denver Developmental Screening Test (DDST)

The Denver Developmental Screening Test (Buros 1971, Frankenburg et al. 1971, Frankenburg et al. 1975) has gained popularity largely through use in preschool programs. The test was designed to be of practical use to untrained evaluators in assessing delayed development in children ages 0 to 6 years. Its design results in a test that is simple, quick to administer, and inexpensive. It assesses development in four areas:

1.   Gross motor: sitting, walking, broad jumping, pedaling a tricycle, throwing a ball overhand, catching a bounced ball, hopping, and balancing on one foot
2.   Fine motor-adaptive: stacking blocks, reaching for objects, drawing a person
3.   Language: responding to a bell, imitating speech sounds, recognizing colors
4.   Personal-social: dressing and smiling responsively

The Denver Developmental Screening Test contains 105 items, but usually no more than 20 items are administered. Each child is tested individually, and performances are rated as normal, abnormal, and questionable for each general area. Each test item is rated according to a developmental "bar" on the record form (Figure 6.1). This scale shows a range of ages by month during which a particular behavior could appear. If a student achieves what 90 percent of the children of that age can achieve on a particular test item, the student "passes." The student would be "delayed" on those items for which she or he did not achieve compared with age peers. Students who display delays in two or more items in a general area are considered "developmentally delayed" in that area.

The test has been criticized for being unrepresentative because of its standardization sample. It was standardized primarily on white children from families of certain occupations that are not reflective of the census distribution. Reliability of the test has also been criticized. Subsequent studies of test-retest and interrater reliabilities revealed less than desirable reliability coefficients (Frankenburg et al. 1971). Her-

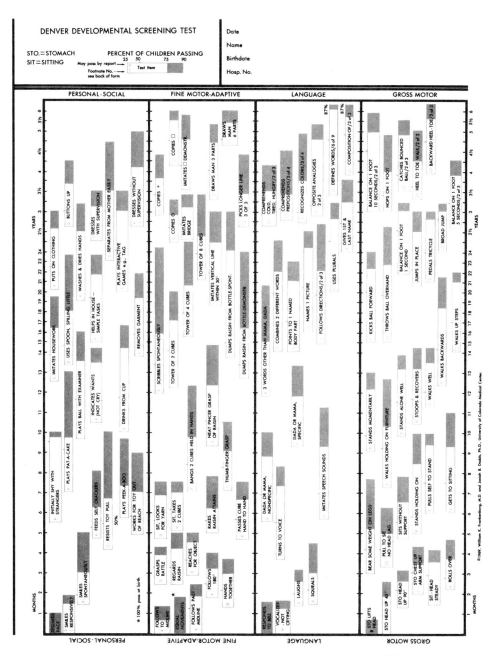

Figure 6.1. Form from Denver Developmental Screening Test (DDST), 1975.

kowitz (1978) reports that the test is only slightly more reliable than information obtained from an interview of the mother.

An evaluation of the validity of the Denver Developmental Screening Test reveals difficulties in diagnosing children less than 30 months old (Herkowitz 1978). Because of criticisms of the test's standardization, reliability, and validity, test users should use the instrument with considerable caution. Whereas the test should not be used for children under 30 months, it is considered acceptable as a screening tool for 4-year-old children. Although the test yields general comparative developmental information, it is of relatively little assistance in instructional planning.

Bayley Scales of Infant Development (BSID)

This developmental test (Bayley 1969, p. 4) is designed to "provide the basis for establishing a child's current status, and thus the extent of any deviation from normal expectancy." The instrument provides three categories of developmental information about children 2 months to $2\frac{1}{2}$ years of age: the Mental Scale, the Motor Scale, and the Infant Behavior Record. In this text we will review the Motor Scale only.

The Motor Scale contains 81 items that measure body control, large muscle coordination, and finger manipulation. Items include progressions such as sitting, standing, walking, climbing stairs, and grasping objects. The results of administering the Motor Scale are expressed as a standard score, the Psychomotor Development Index (PDI).

The Bayley Scales of Infant Development is reported to be well standardized on a sample of 1262 children. Reliability reports on the test reveal relatively low test-retest and tester-observer coefficients on the Motor Scale items that require the tester's assistance (Bayley 1969, Buros 1971). The Motor Scale also has fewer items than the Mental Scale, which results in lower reliability coefficients according to Bayley (1969). No validity information is available on the Motor Scale.

Although the test has a clearly written manual, it is somewhat difficult to administer. The tester has the task of locating the most difficult test items the child can pass. The test takes about 45 minutes to administer (Mental and Motor Scales). The scoring of items is relatively simple, with subsequent conversions to the Psychomotor Development Index. In contrast to the Denver Developmental Screening Test, the Bayley Scales of Infant Development is a more expensive test requiring the construction of some special equipment such as a walking board and a staircase. Because of low reliabilities of Motor Scale items and the lack of validity data, the test should be used with extreme caution.

Gesell Developmental Schedules (GDS)

This instrument (Gesell and Amatruda 1949) compares a list of the child's behaviors with schedules of developmental maturity. It is used most frequently by professionals to assess the development of infants with complications at birth. It also has been used as a predictor of intellectual development in early childhood (4 weeks to 6 years). The Gesell Developmental Schedules provides developmental information in four areas: motor, adaptive, language, and personal-social. The child's behaviors are compared with the age-level constellations of behaviors in the schedules. The test is individually administered in a standard order. One disadvantage of the instrument is that it is expensive, due in part to the dispersion of vital test information in three different volumes.

The Gesell Developmental Schedules was standardized 30 years ago and should be restandardized on today's children. Scant information is available on test reliability. Buros (1965) stresses the need for both test-retest and intertester reliability data. A variety of validity studies have, however, been conducted, and these reveal low predictive validity and high concurrent validity. Because of out-of-date standardization data, the lack of reliability data, and the low predictive validity, the schedules should, like the previous scales, be used with considerable caution.

Other Developmental Tests[1]

Although only three developmental tests have been reviewed here, there is reason to believe that developmental tests in general have severe limitations to their use. In any developmental scale the standardization sample, reliability data, and validity information should be carefully examined. Other available developmental tests include

1. Lincoln-Oseretsky Motor Development Scale (Sloan 1955)
2. Ohio State University Scale of Intra-Gross Motor Assessment (OSU-SIGMA) (Loovis and Ersing 1979).
3. DeOreo Fundamental Motor Skills Inventory (DFMSI) (DeOreo 1976)
4. Milani-Comparetti and Gidoni's Pattern of Analysis of Motor Development (Milani-Comparetti and Gidoni 1967)
5. Apgar's New Method of Evaluation of the Newborn Infant (Apgar 1953)
6. Brazelton's Neonatal Behavioral Assessment Scale (Brazelton 1973)
7. Stott's Test of Motor Impairment (Stott, Moyes, and Henderson 1972)
8. Callier-Azusa Scale (Stillman 1978)
9. Learning Accomplishment Profile (LAP) (Sanford 1975)

Motor Ability Tests

Tests of motor ability are designed to provide comparative information about a student's general motor capabilities or proficiencies. Just as intelligence tests assume that a general index of the construct "intelligence" exists, so motor ability tests assume the existence of a general index for the construct "motor ability." Furthermore, motor ability tests are designed to be predictive of motor skill performance. They are

---

1. A listing of selected motor tests is included in the test index in Appendix A.

usually formal tests standardized on a representative "normal" sample of various age levels. Among the reasons for administering motor ability tests are the following:

1. To determine general motor deficiency
2. To determine motor deficiencies in specific subtest areas
3. To provide empirical data to meet criteria for placement into a developmental/adapted physical education program
4. To determine relative areas of strengths and weaknesses in motor ability
5. To predict success in physical education programs

Some professionals criticize the use of motor ability tests because the tests are not directly related to instructional goals and objectives in physical education. For example, a motor test may identify a student as being "deficient" in "gross body coordination," a so-called underlying motor ability, but the test does not link the result to a physical education objective. The evaluator may well ask, "If Johnny is deficient in gross body coordination, what observable, measurable performance objectives are appropriate for Johnny that fit into the third grade physical education curriculum?" Such questions remain unanswered while physical educators face the dilemma of making sense out of motor ability test results. We recommend that when motor ability tests are used, they be supplemented with locally valid tests of physical education skills. This section includes a review of a commonly used motor ability test, the Bruininks-Oseretsky Test of Motor Proficiency.

The Bruininks-Oseretsky Test of Motor Proficiency (B-O Test)

The Bruininks-Oseretsky Test of Motor Proficiency (Bruininks 1978) is a test of general motor proficiency for children $4^1/_2$ to $14^1/_2$ years of age. An individually administered test, it assesses motor proficiency in gross motor and fine motor areas. The eight subtests include

1. Running speed and agility: measure of speed during a shuttle run
2. Balance: measures static and dynamic balance
3. Bilateral coordination: test of sequential and simultaneous coordination of upper and lower limbs
4. Strength: measures arm-shoulder, abdominal, and leg strength
5. Upper-limb coordination: assesses coordination of visual tracking with arm and hand movements
6. Response speed: measures speed of response to a moving visual stimulus
7. Visual-motor control: assesses the coordination of precise hand and visual movement
8. Upper-limb speed and dexterity: measures hand and finger dexterity, hand and arm speed

The complete test battery provides three estimates of motor ability: a gross motor composite score, a fine motor composite score, and a general index of motor proficiency. For situations such as screening when a brief overview of motor ability is desired, the short form of the test, requiring approximately 20 minutes for administration, can be used.

The complete battery takes about one hour to administer to an individual student. The manual has clearly written directions with illustrations to aid in administration. We recommend that the test be studied and administered by an appropriately trained professional (e.g., developmental/adapted physical educator, occupational therapist). The test is relatively easy to score with guidelines for converting raw scores to percentiles and stanines. Figure 6.2 presents an example of a completed test score summary as it might appear on the student's record form. The most valuable information provided by the test battery is comparative information about the student's general

Complete Battery:

SUBTEST	POINT SCORE Maximum	POINT SCORE Subject's	STANDARD SCORE Test (Table 23)	STANDARD SCORE Composite (Table 24)	PERCENTILE RANK (Table 25)	STANINE (Table 25)	OTHER Age (Equiv.)
GROSS MOTOR SUBTESTS:							
1. Running Speed and Agility	15	8	21				7-8
2. Balance	32	16	13				5-2
3. Bilateral Coordination	20	9	23				7-11
4. Strength	42	5	11				4-11
GROSS MOTOR COMPOSITE			*68 SUM	56	72	6	6-5
5. Upper-Limb Coordination	21	13	*21				6-11
FINE MOTOR SUBTESTS:							
6. Response Speed	17	5	16				6-2
7. Visual-Motor Control	24	18	23				8-5
8. Upper-Limb Speed and Dexterity	72	27	20				6-8
FINE MOTOR COMPOSITE			*59 SUM	64	92	8	6-8
BATTERY COMPOSITE			*148 SUM	63	90	8	6-9

*To obtain Battery Composite: Add Gross Motor Composite, Subtest 5 Standard Score, and Fine Motor Composite. Check result by adding Standard Scores on Subtests 1-8.

Short Form:

	POINT SCORE Maximum	POINT SCORE Subject's	STANDARD SCORE (Table 27)	PERCENTILE RANK (Table 27)	STANINE (Table 27)
SHORT FORM	98				

Figure 6.2. Bruininks-Oseretsky Test of Motor Proficiency test score summary. (From Robert H. Bruininks, *Bruininks-Oseretsky Test of Motor Proficiency.* Circle Pines, Minn.: American Guidance Service, 1978. Reproduced by permission of American Guidance Service.)

motor proficiency relative to his or her age peers. The assessment summary in Figure 6.2 shows how comparative results like percentiles and stanines can be useful in making placement decisions in remedial motor programs.

The Bruininks-Oseretsky Test of Motor Proficiency was standardized on a representative sample of 800 subjects from $4^1/_2$ to $14^1/_2$ years of age. It is one of the first motor tests to be developed from an excellent standardization program. High intercorrelations and high test-retest and interrater reliability coefficients are reported. Validity data presented in the test manual are considered as complete as is possible in an instrument measuring general motor ability. Validity data are also available concerning the test's content and construct validity. Both of Bruininks' studies of contrast groups (1978) reveal the efficiency of the test in discriminating between children with "normal" motor ability and children with motor difficulties. These results support the use of the test for motor screening to identify children with motor difficulties.

Other Motor Ability Tests

In addition to the Bruininks-Oseretsky Test of Motor Proficiency, other tests of general motor ability include

1.   The Project A.C.T.I.V.E. Motor Ability Test (Vodola 1974)
2.   Cratty Six-Category Gross Motor Test (Cratty 1969b)

Physical Fitness Tests

Among all of the physical education tests available, tests of physical fitness are most numerous and are technically most adequate. Physical education teachers are usually familiar with most of the tests. In general, test content is considerably limited. Physical fitness tests measure physical components such as speed, strength, endurance, flexibility, power, and agility. Note that patterns of fundamental motor skills, body management skills, and games and sports skills are usually not evaluated by physical fitness tests. Although fitness tests provide important information about a student's levels of strength, endurance, and flexibility, we recommend that they be supplemented with assessments of other physical education content. This section will review a special physical fitness test that is currently available.

AAHPERD Youth Fitness Test for the Mildly Mentally Retarded

The AAHPERD Special Fitness Test was developed by and is available from the American Alliance for Health, Physical Education, Recreation, and Dance. This special fitness test is designed for students who are mildly mentally retarded and between ages 8 and 18. The AAHPERD Special Fitness Test provides measures of

1.   Arm and shoulder girdle strength (flexed-arm hang)
2.   Efficiency of abdominal and hip flexor muscles (sit-ups)

3. Speed and agility (shuttle run)
4. Explosive muscular power (standing broad jump)
5. Speed (50-yard dash)
6. Skill and coordination (softball throw for distance)
7. Cardiovascular efficiency (300-yard run-walk)

The norms for the AAHPERD Special Fitness Test are based on a standardization sample of 4200 educable mentally retarded boys and girls.

The test is designed to be administered to a class of students (approximately 15 pupils) in about two 30-minute class sessions. Minimal equipment is required, and the test manual is inexpensive. Administration and scoring of the test are straight-forward. Results are reported as percentile scores for each test area. The AAHPERD Special Fitness Test, like the Youth Fitness Test, is associated with a national fitness award system developed to provide recognition to mildly mentally handicapped students for fitness performances.

The test manual does not report reliability and validity data, but this information is available in various studies. Rarick et al. (1976) report substantial test-retest reliability scores. Rarick and Dobbins (1975) obtained high test-retest reliabilities (high .80s and .90s) with educable mentally retarded boys and girls. High validity is claimed because the test measures basic components of children's motor performance (Rarick et al. 1976).

The physical educator is responsible for deciding whether to use a test that has scores compared with a sample of mildly mentally retarded children. A teacher may also choose the Youth Fitness Test if the objective is to compare a handicapped student's performance with "normal" age peers. Other available physical fitness tests[2] are

1. AAHPERD Youth Fitness Test (AAHPERD 1975)
2. AAHPERD Special Fitness Test for Moderately Mentally Retarded Persons (AAHPERD 1976)
3. Physical Fitness Battery for Mentally Retarded Children (Fait 1978)
4. Fleischman Basic Fitness Test (Fleischman 1964)
5. Buell Test (for blind and partially sighted) (Buell 1973)
6. Project Unique (for sensory and orthopedically impaired youth) (Winnick 1979)

Motor Skills Tests

Some physical education tests are designed mainly to assess fundamental motor skills. These tests are primarily criterion-referenced tests that judge a student's per-

---

2. See complete description of selected tests in Appendix A.

formance of a motor skill against some standard (criterion). Skills tests are generally objective-based, measuring a student's progress on a specified performance objective. Because these tests assess observable, measurable motor skills, they usually assess common physical education goals. Some motor skills tests are said to be "curriculum-imbedded," because the student's progress toward objectives is assessed throughout the physical education curriculum. Results of a motor skill test administered to a student with a handicap can be readily translated into individualized education program objectives to meet the mandate of P.L. 94-142. Motor skills tests do not provide comparative data such as percentiles or stanines, but yield instead individualized criterion measurements. One disadvantage of motor skills tests is that they are time consuming because they are usually administered individually on each objective. The primary advantage to motor skills tests is their relevance to physical education instruction. The following section reviews briefly Wessel's *I CAN* program and lists other available motor skills tests.

The *I CAN* Program

The *I CAN* program is a task analyzed, individualized physical education system. The *I CAN* curriculum is a set of diagnostic-prescriptive teaching resource materials with a curriculum structure designed for use with all students. It provides a system for training teachers in planning, assessing, prescribing, teaching, and evaluating student progress in physical education. The program is adaptable to all students, is flexible enough for a variety of settings, is individualized, and is a tool for communication with parents and a management tool for teachers. Means for conducting criterion-referenced assessment and for planning corresponding instructional activities are provided in the following skill areas:

1. Primary skills: fundamental skills, body management, health and fitness, aquatics
2. Secondary skills: Backyard and neighborhood activities, team sports, outdoor activities, dance, and individual sports
3. Preschool skills: locomotor skills, object control skills, play equipment skills, body control skills, participation in play situation skills
4. Associated skills: self-concept, social skills

The *I CAN* method of skill assessment is criterion-referenced to measure a student's current status according to a criterion. The assessment in the *I CAN* program is designed to be administered either individually or to a large group through a specially prepared assessing activity. Children's scores on specific motor skill objectives are marked on a class performance score sheet, which is also used to score progress on objectives. Figure 6.3 shows a sample score sheet.

Advantages of the *I CAN* program and its criterion-referenced assessment are the program's relevance to common physical education objectives, the ease of scoring, and ability to score continuous progress. Disadvantages of the program include lack of comparative test data (percentiles), lack of reliability and validity information, the

I CAN											CLASS PERFORMANCE SCORE SHEET PERFORMANCE OBJECTIVE: OVERHAND THROW	

SCORING — Assessment: X = Achieved, O = Not achieved. Reassessment: ⊗ = Achieved, ⊘ = Not achieved.

FOCAL POINTS / STD.:
- a — Overhand Motion — 10 ft. distance, 2/3 times
- b — Ball Release
- a — Eyes on Target — 20 ft. target at 15 ft., 2/3 times
- b — Overhand Motion
- a — Arm Exten./Side Orient.
- b — Weight Transfer — 2/3 times.
- c — Hip and Spine Rotation
- d — Follow Through
- e — Smooth Integration
- 4 — Angle of Release 45° — age/sex norm., 2/3 times
- 5 — Accuracy — 8 ft. target at 50 ft., 2/3 times
- Primary Responses

PRIMARY RESPONSES: N – Nonattending; NR – No response; UR – Unrelated response; O – Other (specify in comments)

NAME	a	b	a	b	a	b	c	d	e	4	5	COMMENTS
1. John J.	⊗	X	⊗	⊗	⊘	⊗	⊗	⊘	⊘	⊘	⊘	Throws side arm
2. Katie	X	X	X	X	⊗	⊗	⊗	X	⊘	⊘	⊘	
3. Susan	X	X	X	X	X	X	X	X	X	X	⊘	Practice accuracy
4. Mark	X	X	X	X	⊘	X	⊘	⊗	⊘	⊘	⊘	Faces target
5. John S.	X	X	X	X	X	X	X	⊗	⊘	⊘	⊘	Follow through inconsistent
6. Scott	⊗	X	⊘	⊗	⊘	⊘	⊘	⊘	⊘	⊘	⊘	Throws underhand
7. Judy	X	X	⊘	X	⊘	⊘	⊘	⊘	⊘	⊘	⊘	Doesn't look at target
8. Cindy	X	X	X	X	⊗	X	⊗	X	⊘	⊘	⊘	Faces target
9. Kirk	X	X	X	X	X	X	X	X	⊘	⊘	⊘	Jerky
10. Joanie	X	X	X	X	X	⊗	⊗	X	⊘	⊘	⊘	
11. Larry	X	X	X	X	⊗	X	X	X	⊘	⊘	⊘	Arm Bent
12. Chuck	X	X	⊗	⊗	⊘	⊗	⊘	⊘	⊘	⊘	⊘	Throws underhand or side arm unless assisted
13. Linda	X	X	X	X	X	X	X	X	⊗	⊗	⊘	Nearly mature
14. Sherry	X	X	X	X	⊗	X	⊗	X	⊗	⊘	⊘	Inconsistent beginning position
15. Greg	X	X	X	X	X	X	X	X	⊗	⊗	⊗	Nearly mature

Figure 6.3. *I CAN* score sheet. FROM *I CAN Primary Skills*, Janet A. Wessel, Director. Reprinted with permission of the publisher, HUBBARD.

time it takes to assess each objective, and relatively high financial cost. Note also that *I CAN* is based on task analyses of mature patterns of movement and is not developmentally based. *I CAN* assessment is therefore more relevant to instructional planning than to screening or placement.

The *I CAN* assessment materials are most useful for elementary physical education teachers and for physical education teachers of mild, moderate, and severely handicapped students. The leisure and recreation assessment materials would probably be most useful with secondary school students with handicaps and with adult handicapped students.

Other Motor Skills Tests[3] include

1. Godfrey-Kephart Movement Pattern Checklist—Short Form (Godfrey and Kephart 1969)
2. Project A.C.T.I.V.E. criterion-referenced skill assessments (Vodola 1974)
3. John Dunn's Data Based Physical Education (Dunn 1980)
4. Preschool Recreation Enrichment Program (PREP)
5. Brigance Diagnostic Inventory of Early Development (Motor Skills Portions) (Brigance 1978)

Perceptual-Motor Tests

Many perceptual-motor tests were developed in the mid-1960s and the 1970s. Perceptual-motor tests were popular among practitioners in the field of learning disabilities. The basic assumption underlying these tests is that academic learning difficulties can be remedied through perceptual-motor activities. This premise has since been refuted by such research experts as Salvia and Ysseldyke (1981, p. 367) who report

> The practice of perceptual-motor assessment is linked directly to perceptual-motor training or remediation. There is a tremendous lack of empirical evidence to support the claim that specific perceptual-motor training facilitates the acquisition of academic skills or improves the chances of academic success. Perceptual-motor training will improve *perceptual-motor* functioning. When the purpose of perceptual-motor assessment is to identify specific important perceptual and motor behaviors that children have not yet mastered, some of the devices . . . may provide useful information; performance on individual items will indicate the extent to which specific skills (for example, walking along a straight line) have been mastered. There is no support for the use of perceptual-motor tests in planning programs designed to facilitate academic learning or remediate academic difficulties.

Perceptual-motor tests have made contributions, however, to the field of adapted physical education. The assumption underlying the application of perceptual-motor theory in adapted physical education programs is that all motor activities possess some component of perceptual-motor functioning. By assessing and providing training in perceptual-motor skills, teachers are assuming that these skills will transfer and generalize to functional movement skills. The assumption of transfer of training remains debatable, while more criterion-referenced motor skills tests gain in popularity. We will review the Purdue Perceptual-Motor Survey and list other available perceptual-motor tests.

---

3. A more detailed description of selected tests can be found in Appendix A.

The Purdue Perceptual-Motor Survey (PPMS)

The Purdue Perceptual-Motor Survey (Roach and Kephart 1966, p. 2) was designed to assess "qualitatively the perceptual-motor abilities of children in the early grades." The test measures perceptual-motor performance in five areas: balance and posture, body image and differentiation, ocular control, form perception, and perceptual-motor matching. These five areas are assessed by 11 subtests that include 22 scorable items. Roach and Kephart (1966, p. 11) state that the test was not designed to diagnose, but "to allow the clinician to observe perceptual-motor behavior in a series of behavioral performances."

The survey is designed to be administered individually to children, age 6 to 10, who do not have specific sensory or physical disabilities such as blindness, paralysis, or physical impairments. The behaviors sampled in the five areas include the following:

1. Balance and posture: walking a balance beam and jumping
2. Body image and differentiation: identification of body parts, imitation of movement, obstacle course, Kraus-Weber, and "angels in the snow"
3. Perceptual-motor match: drawing a circle, drawing two circles simultaneously, drawing a lateral line, and drawing two straight lines vertically simultaneously
4. Ocular control: movement of eyes following a flashlight, and convergence on objects
5. Form perception: copying seven geometric forms

The scoring procedures for the survey are primarily qualitative and subjective. An example of the record form is shown in Figure 6.4. The form is essentially a checklist that notes specific difficulties on each of the items.

Standardization of the Purdue Perceptual-Motor Survey was conducted on 200 children, age 6 to 10, who were known to be free of motor difficulties. The test authors report a test-retest reliability of .95, based on scores of 30 children from the standardization sample. We have little validity information that the survey tests what it purports to measure. The instrument should be used cautiously and be supplemented with other assessment information of physical education performance.

Other Perceptual-Motor Tests[4] are

1. Cratty Six-Category Gross Motor Test (Cratty 1969b)
2. Frostig Developmental Test of Visual Perception (Frostig and Whittlesey 1966)
3. Southern California Test of Sensory Integration (Ayres 1980)

---

4. A more detailed description of selected tests is included in Appendix A.

Perceptual-Motor Survey

Name _Jane Doe_ Date of birth _9/19/53_
Address _1321 E. 23rd. St._ Sex _F_ Grade _3_
Homewood School _Central_
Examiner _J. H._ Date of examination _6/16/64_

	4	3	2	1	
Walking Board: Forward		X			Balance and Posture
Backward			X		
Sidewise				X	
Jumping		X			Body Image and Differentiation
Identification of Body Parts	X				
Imitation of Movement		X			
Obstacle Course			X		
Kraus-Weber	X				
Angels-in-the-snow			X		
Chalkboard Circle			X		Perceptual-Motor Match
Double Circle				X	
Lateral Line			X		
Vertical Line		X			
Rhythmic writing Rhythm				X	
Reproduction			X		
Orientation				X	
Ocular Pursuits Both eyes			X		Ocular Control
Right eye				X	
Left eye				X	
Convergence			X		
Visual Achievement Forms Form				X	Form Perception
Organization		X			

Figure 6.4. Purdue Perceptual-Motor Survey record form (Roach and Kephart 1966).

Behavioral Tests

Most educators would agree that behavior and participation in group activities are among the most difficult areas to assess. The measurement of group participation is usually provided through the use of informal tests of behavior such as checklists and rating scales. Participation assessment may involve an assessment of both social interaction and cognitive "style" in the physical education setting. Behavioral assessment is gaining increasing popularity as a meaningful data base for effecting behavior change. Several key generalizations (adapted from Mash and Terdal 1976) are characteristic of behavioral assessment:

1. The physical education setting is a controlled setting in which antecedents, behaviors, and consequences are easily defined.
2. Measurement must include forms of environmental stimulation (e.g., bright lights or loud noises) that are present while the behavior is occurring. Development of an instrument to describe situational variables is a needed refinement in the field.
4. Focus of assessment is on providing information that can be used to design, implement, and evaluate programs.
5. Assessment should replicate naturally occurring conditions.
6. Assessment is ongoing and self-corrective. Measurement is repeated on a consistent, time-sampling basis.
7. Assessment is not oriented toward pathology but toward situation-specific strengths, assets, and deficiencies.

Behavioral assessment depends on accurate observation and precise measurement. It is, therefore, important for physical educators to define precisely the behaviors they are about to assess and be prepared to accurately observe and record them. Behavioral assessment in physical education can be used to do the following:

1. Screen for behavior problems
2. Define and quantify motor behavior problems
3. Pinpoint and design intervention
4. Monitor progress
5. Follow-up

This section will review one behavioral assessment method and suggest other available behavior tests.

Walker Problem Behavior Identification Checklist (WPBIC)

The checklist (Walker 1976) is a standardized norm-referenced assessment designed to identify students with possible behavior problems. It was developed to be used by teachers with students in the fourth, fifth, and sixth grades. Although designed for classroom use, the checklist can also be useful in physical education settings. It measures five areas of behavior with 50 items. The behavior areas are (1) acting out, (2) withdrawal, (3) distractibility, (4) disturbed peer relations, and (5) immaturity. The checklist can be completed in as little time as 5 minutes. Sample items include

Habitually rejects the school experience through actions or comments
Has temper tantrums
Does not obey until threatened with punishment
Reacts with defiance to instructions or commands
Does not engage in group activities
Is overactive, restless, or continually shifting body positions
Utters nonsense syllables or babbles to himself or herself or does both

The Walker Problem Behavior Identification Checklist was standardized on 534 children in grades four, five, and six. Validity information includes data on criterion validity, factorial validity, and item validity. The reported reliability coefficient is .98.

The checklist should be supplemented with other behavioral assessment data to provide a picture of motor behavior as well as "acting out" behavior. Other behavioral tests[5] include

1. Burks' Behavior Rating Scales (BBRS) (Burks 1977)
2. Child Behavior Rating Scale (CBRS) (Cassel 1978)

Leisure Recreation Assessment

The ultimate goal in physical education is to ensure a lifetime of health and wellness by providing the necessary skills and experiences to incorporate regular enjoyable physical activity into each person's adult life. While many would agree with this goal, an important area of physical education that is overlooked is leisure and recreation. In adapted physical education, assessment and programming that include objectives of leisure and recreation are consequently scarce. A comprehensive assessment in adapted physical education should include the assessment of leisure and recreational skills, participation, and preferences. While components of leisure and recreation should be assessed and programmed at all ages, there should be increased emphasis on leisure and recreation programming in secondary level programs (ages 12 to 21). Wehman and Schleien (1981) proposed that a teacher should ask questions before making decisions about assessment and instruction. Such questions might include

Preference   What skills does the student already
                              demonstrate?
Functioning   What are the student's capabilities
                              and educational needs?

---

5. Selected motor assessment tests are described in Appendix A.

Physical characteristics

What physical characteristics does the student have or lack that may interfere with leisure skills development?

Age appropriateness

Are the skills that have been selected for instruction the type of skills that nonhandicapped age peers might engage in?

Access to materials

What is the student's access to materials (e.g., financial resources, transportation)?

Support of home environment

What persons are available in the home or neighborhood environments to reinforce leisure skills development?

One type of leisure assessment is a leisure skill inventory, which measures a student's leisure and recreation skill levels. Leisure skill inventories are primarily criterion-referenced instruments, or simple task analyses of leisure skills. Wehman and Schleien (1981) suggest an example of a task analysis for tossing a Frisbee (Figure 6.5). This behavioral method of assessment provides a continuous record of progress as

Task Analytic Assessment for Tossing a Frisbee					
Step	M	T	W	Th	F
1. Extend hand downward toward Frisbee.	+	+	+	+	+
2. Curl fingers underneath Frisbee.	+	+	+	+	+
3. Position thumb on top edge of Frisbee.	+	+	−	+	+
4. Apply inward pressure with fingers and thumb to grasp Frisbee firmly.	−	−	−	+	+
5. Bend at elbow, raising Frisbee to chest.	−	−	−	−	−
6. Hold Frisbee parallel to ground.	−	−	−	−	−
7. Bring Frisbee inward toward nondominant side of body.	−	−	−	−	−
8. Quickly extend elbow outward away from body.	−	−	−	−	−
9. Snap wrist outward and extend fingers to release Frisbee.	−	−	−	−	−
10. Toss Frisbee 2 feet.	−	−	−	−	−
11. Toss Frisbee 3 feet.	−	−	−	−	−
12. Toss Frisbee 4 feet.	−	−	−	−	−
13. Toss Frisbee 5 feet.	−	−	−	−	−

Figure 6.5. Example of a task analytic assessment (Wehman and Schleien 1981).

well as a measurement of entry level of performance.

The *I CAN* program (Wessel 1979) provides sport, leisure, and recreation curricular materials for backyard or neighborhood activities, team sports, outdoor activities, dance, and individual sports. As in the primary skills section of the *I CAN* program, the sport, leisure, and recreation materials include a task analysis assessment of each skill.

Other methods of leisure assessment include measuring the level of participation in leisure activities, which may include measuring the student's attention to the activity, the appropriateness of the student's behaviors, and the student's levels of social interaction.

In order to prepare a student to make leisure and recreational choices as an adult, the evaluator may wish to assess the student's leisure preferences. Knowledge of the student's activity choices can help motivation, development of the individualized education program, and the teaching of prerequisite skills.

References

AAHPERD. *Special Fitness Test Manual for Mildly Mentally Retarded Persons.* Reston, VA: The Alliance, 1976.

AAHPERD. *Youth Fitness Test Manual.* Reston, VA: The Alliance, 1975.

Apgar, V. A Proposal for the New Method of Evaluation of the Newborn Infant. *Current Research in Anesthesiology* 32:260–70, 1953.

Ayres, A. J. *Southern California Sensory Integration Tests.* Los Angeles: Western Psychological Services, 1980.

Bayley, N. A. The Development of Motor Abilities during the First Three Years. *Society for Research in Child Development* 1:1–26, 1935.

Bayley, N. A. *Manual for the Bayley Scales of Infant Development.* New York: The Psychological Corporation, 1969.

Brazelton, T. B. *Neonatal Behavioral Assessment Scale.* Clinics in Developmental Medicine, No. 50, Philadelphia, PA: Spastics International Publications, Lippincott, 1973.

Brigance, A. *Brigance Diagnostic Inventory of Basic Skills.* North Billerica, MA: Curriculum Associates, 1977.

Brigance, A. *Brigance Diagnostic Inventory of Early Development.* North Billerica, MA: Curriculum Associates, 1978.

Brigance, A. *Brigance Diagnostic Inventory of Essential Skills.* North Billerica, MA: Curriculum Associates, 1980.

Bruininks, R. H. *Bruininks-Oseretsky Test of Motor Proficiency.* Circle Pines, MN: American Guidance Service, 1978.

Buell, C. *Physical Education and Recreation for the Visually Handicapped.* Washington, DC: American Association for Health, Physical Education, and Recreation, 1973.

Burks, H. F. *Burks' Behavior Rating Scales.* Los Angeles: Western Psychological Services, 1969, rev. ed., 1977.

Buros, O. K., ed. *The Sixth Mental Measurements Yearbook.* Highland Park, NJ: Gryphon Press, 1965.

Buros, O. K., ed. *The Seventh Mental Measurements Yearbook.* Highland Park, NJ: Gryphon Press, 1971, entry 405.

Buros, O. K., ed. *The Eighth Annual Mental Measurements Yearbook (Vols. 1 and 2).* Highland Park, NJ: Gryphon Press, 1978.

Cassel, R. H. *The Child Behavior Rating Scale.* Los Angeles: Western Psychological Services, 1978.

Cratty, B. J. *Motor Activity and the Education of Retardates.* Philadelphia, PA: Lea & Febiger, 1969a.

Cratty, B. J. *Perceptual-Motor Behavior and Educational Processes.* Springfield, IL: Charles C. Thomas, 1969b.

Cratty, B. J. Adapted Physical Education for Handicapped Children and Youth. Denver, CO: Love, 1980.

DeOreo, K. L. Unpublished current work on the assessment of the development of gross motor skills. Kent State University, 1976.

Dunn, J. M. et al. *A Data Based Gymnasium: A Systematic Approach to Physical Education for the Handicapped.* Instructional Development Corporation, Monmouth, OR, 1980.

Fait, H. *Physical Fitness Battery for Mentally Retarded Children.* Storrs, CT: School of Physical Education, University of Connecticut, 1978.

Fleischman, E. W. *The Structure and Measurement of Physical Fitness.* Englewood Cliffs, NJ: Prentice-Hall, 1964.

Frankenburg, W., Goldstein, A., and Camp, B. The Revised Denver Developmental Screening Test: Its Accuracy as a Screening Instrument. *Pediatrics* 79:988–995, 1971.

Frankenburg, W. K. et al. *Denver Developmental Screening Test, Reference Manual, Revised 1975 Edition.* Denver, CO: LADOCA Project Publishing Foundation, 1975.

Frankenburg, W. K. et al. Reliability and Stability of the Denver Developmental Screening Test. *Child Development* 42:1315–1325, 1971.

Frostig, M., Lefeber, W., and Whittlesey, J. *Administration and Scoring Manual for the Marianne Frostig Developmental Test of Visual Perception.* Palo Alto, CA: Consulting Psychologists Press, 1966.

Gesell, A., and Amatruda, C. S. *Gesell Developmental Schedules.* New York: Psychological Company, 1949.

Godfrey, B. B., and Kephart, N. C. *Movement Patterns and Motor Education.* New York: Appleton-Century Crofts, 1969.

Herkowitz, J. Assessing the Motor Development of Children: Presentation and Critique of Tests. In M. Ridenour (ed.) *Motor Development.* Princeton, NJ: Princeton Book Company, 1978.

Kelso, S., and Clark, J. *The Development of Movement Control and Coordination.* New York: Wiley, 1982.

Loovis, M. Model for Individualizing Physical Education Experiences for the Preschool Moderately Retarded Child. (Doctoral dissertation, The Ohio State University, 1975). Dissertation Abstracts International, 1976, 36 5126A (University Microfilms No. 76-3485).

Loovis, M., and Ersing, W. F. Ohio State University SIGMA, in Assessing and Programming Gross Motor Development for Children. Cleveland Heights, OH: Ohio Motor Assessment Associates, 1979.

Mash, E., and Terdal, L. *Behavior Therapy Assessment.* New York: Springer, 1976.

Milani-Comparetti, A., and Gidoni, E. A Pattern Analysis of Motor Development and its Disorders. *Developmental Medicine and Child Neurology* 11:625–30, 1967.

Preschool Recreation Enrichment Program (PREP). Washington, DC: Hawkins and Associates.

Rarick, G. L., and Dobbins, D. A. Basic Components in the Motor Performance of Children From Six to Nine Years. *Medicine and Science in Sports* 7:105–110, 1975.

Rarick, G. L., Dobbins, D. A., and Broadhead, G. D. *The Motor Domain and Its Correlates in Educationally Handicapped Children.* Englewood Cliffs, NJ: Prentice-Hall, 1976.

Roach, E. F., and Kephart, N. C. *The Purdue Perceptual-Motor Survey.* Columbus, OH: Charles E. Merrill, 1966.

Salvia, J., and Ysseldyke, J. *Assessment in Special and Remedial Education.* Boston: Houghton Mifflin, 1981.

Sanford, A. *The Learning Accomplishment Profile.* Winston-Salem, NC: Kaplan School Supply, 1975.

Sloan, W. The Lincoln-Oseretsky Motor Development Scale. *Genetic Psychology Monographs* 51:183–252, 1955.

Stillman, R., ed. *The Callier-Azusa Scale.* Washington, DC: U.S. Office of Education, No. 300750289, 1978.

Stott, D. H., Moyes, F. A., and Henderson, S. E. *Test of Motor Impairment.* Guelph, Ontario: Brook Educational Publishing, 1972.

Vodola, T. M., *All Children Totally Involved Exercising.* Oakhurst, NJ: Township of Ocean School District, 1974.

Walker, H. M. *Walker Problem Behavior Identification Checklist.* (rev. ed.) Los Angeles: Western Psychological Services, 1976.

Wehman, P., and Schleien, S. *Leisure Programs for Handicapped Persons.* Baltimore, MD: University Park Press, 1981.

Wessel, J. A., Project Director. *I CAN: Primary Skills.* Northbrook, IL: Hubbard, 1976.

Wessel, J. A., Project Director. *I CAN: Sport, Leisure and Recreation Skills.* Northbrook, IL: Hubbard, 1980.

Winnick, J., and Silva, J. *Project Unique: The Physical Fitness and Performance of Sensory and Orthopedically Impaired Youth.* State University of New York, College at Brockport, NY, 1979.

CHAPTER 7

Translating Assessment
Into Action: A Team Approach

Information gathered about a student's physical education performance, motor proficiency, or level of physical fitness can provide an interesting description about a student's psychomotor skill level. This array of information is of little use, however, unless the data are interpreted and communicated meaningfully by the tester. It is this next step, after the assessment is completed, that will have an important impact on the physical education programming decisions for students with handicaps. The general purpose of the adapted physical education assessment is not to diagnose disabilities or diseases but to plan appropriate programs. The challenge confronting the adapted physical educator as a member of a child study team is to translate into action the data gathered from observing the student and administering tests. This chapter will present guidelines for (1) the preparation and interpretation of assessment data, (2) the interactions and roles of members of the individualized education program (IEP) team, (3) the writing of adapted physical education goals and objectives, (4) making decisions about instructional activities, and (5) establishing procedures for periodic review and evaluation of progress.

Preparation and Interpretation of Assessment Information

Assuming that a comprehensive assessment of physical education performance has been completed, the tester will be faced with data in varying forms. An informal test of physical education behavior may yield data consisting of summaries of observation tallies. A standardized test will yield raw scores, percentiles, and stanines, and a developmental profile may result in developmental ages. The physical educator's challenge is summarizing and drawing conclusions from this "bank" of data that have been gathered and summarized in different forms. Before the information can be translated into instruction, the tester should take care to prepare the data for interpretation.

Preparing the Data

Whether the results of the assessment are to be presented verbally or in written form, the tester must proceed systematically to present a cohesive picture of the student's psychomotor performance. As the test information is being interpreted, the following assessment components should be recorded and prepared for summary and interpretation.

1. Demographic data: Include the student's full name, birthdate, grade placement, address, telephone number, classroom teacher, and case manager (primary special education teacher, if appropriate).
2. Referral data: Include the name of the person who initiated the referral, the referral date, and the reason for referral.
3. Background data: May include information from physicians, therapists, parents, and others concerning the student's physical, educational, and sociocultural background and status.
4. Observational data noted during assessment: Notes and comments about the student's behavior during the assessment sessions should be recorded.
5. Test data: All assessment data should be tallied and summarized in raw score form to prepare for further analysis and interpretation.

It is important that the tester review the completed student response forms for a final check to be certain that the data have been recorded properly. At this point, the evaluator should choose only the relevant data for reporting and interpreting. The student's privacy rights are violated when irrelevant information (i.e., reading achievement scores, family socioeconomic status) is used in the decision-making process.

Summarizing Formal Test Data

Several methods are available to expedite the process of summarizing a vast array of test data on an individual student. The goal in summarizing test data is to describe the student's physical education strengths and needs in a concise form to facilitate both communication and decision making. Informal and formal assessment data of the highest quality should first be summarized as raw scores. Note, however, that raw scores by themselves are of extremely limited value. If a formal, standardized test has been administered, the raw scores need to be converted to other types of scores. This conversion allows the student's scores to be compared with scores achieved by students in the standardization population. Raw scores may also be converted to derived scores such as age-equivalent scores, grade-equivalent scores, percentiles, standard scores, and stanines. Generally a tester can convert raw scores to other scores by using tables provided in the test manual. Derived scores include:

1. Age-equivalent scores: Raw scores are translated into the average chronological age (CA) at which the students in the standardization population achieved a particular raw score. For example, Katy, whose CA is 10.3, achieved an age-equivalent score of 5.11 on a bilateral coordination subtest. Katy's motor performance on this test was like that of students age 5 years 11 months, revealing a problem area for a child age 10.

2. Grade-equivalent scores: Raw scores are translated into the average grade at which students in the standardization population achieved a particular raw score. For example, John, who is at the beginning of third grade, achieved a grade-equivalent score of 1.5 (based on a raw score of 6) on an abdominal strength subtest. This means that the average grade-equivalent score in the standardization group that received a raw score of 6 on the subtest was grade 1.5, indicating grade one and five-tenths.

3. Percentiles: Most standardized tests provide tables for the conversion of raw scores to percentile ranks. A percentile rank indicates the percentage of students in the standardization group that received the same raw score or a lower raw score. For example, if Lisa, age eight, achieved a raw score of 14 in running speed and agility, the corresponding percentile rank in the test norms might be the 35th percentile. This means that a raw score of 14 is equal to or higher than the scores achieved by 35 percent of the standardization group. Lisa obtained a score higher than 35 out of every 100 students in a representative sample of eight-year-olds. Percentile ranks are commonly used in IEP team meetings for reporting test results, because they are fairly easy to calculate and interpret.

4. Standard scores: In standardized tests, raw scores are usually converted to standard scores before further conversions to percentiles and stanines are made. Standard scores provide a scale of scores that can be used for comparisons of all students to whom the test was administered. The mean and the standard deviation are used to calculate standard scores, which are usually presented in the norm tables of the test manual. The mean ($\bar{X}$) of a set of scores is the arithmetic average, and is usually presented in motor test manuals for students of different ages. The standard deviation (SD) of a set of scores describes the variability of the scores. For example, Todd, when compared with his age peers, achieved a standard score of 40 on a motor ability test. Since the mean standard score on this test is 50 and the standard deviation is 10, Todd's score indicates that his performance was one standard deviation below the mean of the norm group for Todd's age.

5. Stanines: Some standardized tests allow the tester to convert raw scores to stanines. Stanines are simply ranges of standard scores. The use of stanines has become increasingly popular in public schools for interpreting and describing formal test results. There are nine stanines, or "standard nines." One advantage in using stanine scores is that collapsing the full range of standard scores into nine categories helps guard against over-interpretation of test data, particularly when differences between students' scores are slight. The con-

version of raw scores into stanines is usually provided in tables in the test manual.

Derived scores such as percentiles, standard scores, and stanines provide a means for comparing one individual's raw scores with a "normal distribution" of raw scores. The standardization sample reported in the test manual has raw scores that are distributed normally in a bell-shaped curve. (Figure 5.7 shows the relationship of derived scores to the normal distribution.)

When a formal, standardized test has been administered and raw scores converted to derived scores, a student's test scores may be plotted on a profile. A test profile is the visual presentation of a student's test performance, and is often useful in interpreting test results to parents and other team members. Figure 7.1 presents a sample test profile for a student who was administered the Bruininks-Oseretsky Test of Motor Proficiency. A brief study of a student's test profile allows the tester, team members, and parents to ascertain quickly the student's motor strengths and weaknesses. Profiles can be of assistance in program planning, but should be used in conjunction with other psychomotor assessment methods and summaries when vital educational decisions are being made.

Summarizing Informal Test Data

When interviews, observational checklists, and criterion-referenced assessment methods are used, the form of the test data is frequently more qualitative than quantitative. Such methods compare a student to a criterion rather than to scores of age peers. Although informal assessment methods have the advantage of being immediately applicable to the understanding and solution of relevant problems in physical education, the results are often difficult to interpret. Some informal measures do include a criterion for motor performance, but those criteria are subjectively established.

To assist in summarizing informal test information, we recommend that results be depicted in graphic form. For example, in the *I CAN* program (Wessel 1976), physical education skills are task analyzed. Assessment and recording of *I CAN* skills simply allows the tester to check whether a specific component (focal point) of a skill has been achieved. If not, IEP objectives can easily be written for areas in which improvement is needed as indicated on a summary profile (Figure 7.2). If information describing motor behavior has been gathered by means of an observation checklist (Figure 7.3), the data can be summarized on a graph. (Checks for reliability and objectivity should be completed prior to assessment.) The derived levels of mastery for the student's age or grade level must also be recorded. A student's strengths and needs should be readily apparent through a brief examination of a graph.

Because an adapted physical educator will probably have accumulated assessment data in varying forms, a comprehensive summary listing the student's strengths and needs should be compiled. Figure 7.4 presents a summary of the areas of instructional need for a student, Alice, based on four different assessment instruments. Each "test" contributed valuable information that was essential to arriving at a complete picture of Alice's skill difficulties. While the summary in Figure 7.4 does not indicate the

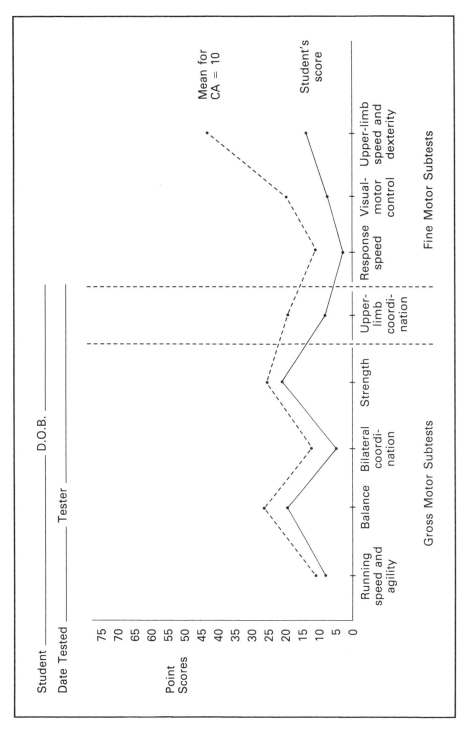

Figure 7.1. Sample Bruininks-Oseretsky Test of Motor Proficiency student profile.

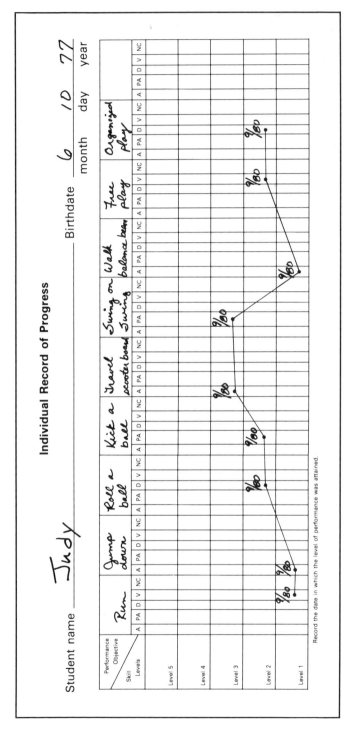

Figure 7.2. A sample preschool student profile from the I CAN program (Wessel 1980). From I CAN Sport, Leisure and Recreation Skills, Janet A. Wessel, Director. Reprinted with permission of the publisher, HUBBARD.

P.E. Skills		9-27	10-1	10-4	10-8	10-15	X̄ Score
Balance		0	0	1	0	1	.4
Run		2	3	2	2	2	2.2
Gallop		1	2	1	2	2	1.6
High jump	Locomotor	2	1	1	1	2	1.4
Vertical jump		2	2	1	1	2	1.6
Hop		1	0	2	1	1	1.0
Skip		0	0	0	0	1	.2
Catch		1	1	2	2	2	1.6
Chest pass	Object Control	2	2	2	2	2	2.0
Underhand throw		1	1	1	1	1	1.0
Overhand throw		1	1	1	1	1	1.0
Kick		1	2	2	1	1	.4
Rope jump	Bilat. Coord.	0	0	0	1	1	.4
Jumping jacks		1	1	1	1	1	1.0
Curl-ups		1	1	2	1	1	1.2
Seal walk	Fitness	0	0	0	0	0	.0
Endurance		2	2	2	2	2	2.0
Dodging		1	1	1	2	2	1.4
Start/stop		1	1	2	2	2	1.6

Student __Tom__ D.O.B. __4-9-75__
Grade __2__ Teacher __M. Brown__

Scale: 0–0.75 Unable to perform the skill
0.75–1.50 Rudimentary (poor) performance
1.50–2.25 Functional (average) performance
2.25–3.0 Proficient (excellent) performance

Figure 7.3. Raw test data from observations checklist.

nature of the cause of these difficulties, it does provide vital information for determining the general goals of Alice's IEP. The profiles from individual tests plus a summary of educational needs help communicate assessment results to the child study team. Such summary information also provides an effective means of communicating a student's skill status in physical education to parents.

Areas of Instructional Needs

Student _Alice_

Grade _7_

Disability _Learning disabled_

	AAHPERD Youth Fitness Test	Bruininks-Oseretsky Motor Test	Observation Checklists	I CAN Task Analysis
Fitness	Heart-lung endurance	Speed/agility	Endurance	
General Coordination		Balance Bilateral coord.	Jumping jacks Burpees	
Object Control Skills		Upper-limb coordination	Tennis strike Volleyball serve Soccer kick Soccer dribble	Ball bounce Side-arm strike Underhand strike
Locomotor Skills				
Social Skills			Withdrawn Misses class often Stands in background Quiet	
Cognitive Skills			Difficulty following game strategies	

Figure 7.4. Comprehensive summary of areas of instructional need.

Interpreting Test Results

Once the test data have been gathered and summarized, the tester must interpret the findings and suggest program options for meeting the student's physical education needs. At this point, the tester should have determined the overall level of motor functioning in all areas measured. In addition, the current level of performance in each specific area (i.e., arm strength, static balance, and so forth) should be reported with strengths and weaknesses noted. The tester's challenge is now to examine the student's problem areas and determine (1) their interrelationships, (2) their relationship to the student's handicapping condition, and (3) their impact on performance in physical education and on overall physical functioning.

When studying assessment results, the evaluator should look for patterns or trends among problem areas. Assuming that reliable and valid assessment techniques were used, the tester should note consistencies and inconsistencies in the results. For example, if one test revealed deficits in balance but another assessment demonstrated "average" performance, these inconsistencies should be examined. Another check of reliability and validity may reveal the source of the inconsistencies. Carefully administered tests and assessment methods disclose consistent areas of motor strengths and needs. For example, if one test revealed deficits in upper-limb coordination and if observations of physical education performance showed problems with throwing and catching, the tester could be relatively confident that these areas indeed represent skill discrepancies. In examining test results for interrelationships, one may find that deficits in balance may coincide with problems in agility and body-management skills. Difficulties in locomotor patterns may coexist with problems in bilateral coordination, and low fitness may exist as a sole problem in physical education. Basically, the tester needs to examine the test summaries and to note patterns, trends, and inconsistencies among the data before making recommendations.

While interpreting the test data, the evaluator must study any relationships that may exist among the identified skill problem areas and the student's handicapping condition. The tester could expect, for example, that a student physically handicapped with muscular dystrophy will show deficits in areas of strength, endurance, and locomotor skills. A student who is learning disabled will often have difficulties with eye-hand coordination and balance. In yet another situation, a child with a hearing impairment may perform well in all skill areas but have difficulty following verbal directions. Information gleaned from such relationships can be valuable both in understanding the nature of the student's motor problems and in designing an appropriate IEP. Knowledge about a student's learning problems and cognitive style can help the adapted physical educator select appropriate instructional strategies.

The next question the tester must explore is, "To what degree do these problems influence performance in physical education classes and overall physical functioning?" Answering this question requires professional judgment and a clear picture of all of the intervening variables. Not only must the tester have a thorough understanding of the student's motor strengths and difficulties, but he or she should also understand the student's current physical education environment. Some questions that will be helpful to answer include the following:

1. What is the severity of the deficits in motor performance?
2. In which areas of physical education does the student have special educational needs?
3. What are the teacher's skill development expectations in the student's physical education class?
4. What expectations for physical functioning exist outside the physical education class?

Severity of Discrepancies

In examining the test results, the evaluator should note how discrepant the student's performance is compared with age and grade norms. Standardized tests conveniently provide percentile ranks, stanines, and standard scores to facilitate interpretation. One or more standard deviations below the mean, stanine scores of one, two, or three, and percentile ranks of below 16, all indicate below average performance. Scores closer to the mean, for example, only one or less standard deviations from the mean, indicate potential problems but to a milder degree. Students with severe discrepancies may need special instruction through an adapted physical education program.

When informal assessment results are being interpreted, making decisions about the severity of discrepancies is more complex. In a criterion-referenced assessment, the student's performance has been measured against a criterion. If the student's performance was less than mastery or did not meet the criterion expected for grade level, one must use professional judgment in analyzing the severity of the discrepancy between student performance and criterion. For example, if an *I CAN* assessment was used to evaluate Sarah's overhand throw, and if she achieved level 2b (an immature throwing pattern), the tester must ask some further questions before recommending a program for Sarah.

1. What level of overhand throw should be expected for Sarah given her age, grade level, and disability?
2. Is Sarah's throwing skill at a significantly "lower" level of performance than one could expect for Sarah?

Answering these questions requires a thorough understanding of the student and her skill needs, as well as knowing her physical education environment.

Areas of Physical Education Needs.   While analyzing the results of the assessment, the tester should note how many and which skill areas reveal difficulties. A student who demonstrates deficits in all areas of physical education has a more critical need for special intervention than does a student who has difficulties in only one area. Katy, for example, who showed below average physical fitness levels, may not require as immediate and intensive programming as Timothy, who has difficulties in general coordination, locomotor skills, and object control skills. Although Katy should receive special assistance to improve her fitness levels, programming can be planned to take place within the regular class or at home or in both settings. In contrast,

Timothy's motor needs in so many areas will require a more comprehensive program of special instruction. Depending on the severity of his difficulties, Timothy's program may occur through an adapted physical education class or in special training as a supplement to his regular class. The tester will plan for individual student needs after analyzing the severity and scope of the problems and their interaction.

Skill Expectations in Physical Education

The skill levels needed for successful performance in the student's physical education class should also be carefully considered. For example, a student's regular eighth grade class is based on prerequisite skills for volleyball and soccer, but the handicapped student's assessment results reveal serious difficulties in those prerequisite skills. The tester can be reasonably confident in predicting that the student will struggle with those skills in the regular class. An individualized adapted physical education program can be planned that provides special instruction in prerequisite skill areas while the student participates in the regular class.

Expectations also exist for students who are severely handicapped and have a "gross motor class" as a part of their total physical education program. A task analysis assessment of rudimentary motor skills will reveal areas in which programming should occur. The tester must then decide how to present the programming: in a group setting, on a one-to-one basis, or in a combination of settings.

Expectations for Physical Functioning

Another vital consideration when interpreting assessment results is the expectation of the student for physical functioning in environments outside the physical education class. Recognized levels of physical functioning that can assist in setting IEP goals and objectives are as follows:

1. Physical Functioning Level I: nonambulatory, simple upper-body skills such as reach, grasp, trunk control, and head control
2. Physical Functioning Level II: rudimentary locomotion such as creep, crawl, cruise, stand; basic object manipulation such as grasp, release, throw, push, pull; basic body awareness; motor skills for personal care such as feeding, toileting and dressing, and righting reflexes
3. Physical Functioning Level III: functional patterns of fundamental motor skills such as walk, run, vertical jump, up and down stairs, overhand throw, underhand throw, low to average levels of physical fitness, and basic body awareness and body management; participation in playground activities
4. Physical Functioning Level IV: mature patterns in some fundamental skills of locomotion and object control, good static and dynamic balance, average levels of fitness, may participate in intramural activities or sports or both

The combination of problem severity and scope and classroom expectations for physical functioning should guide the tester in making a professional interpretation of assessment results and in making appropriate recommendations for programming.

Team Decision Making

When results from individualized assessment are brought to the IEP meeting, the meeting purpose is broader than simply presenting the findings. It is, rather, to share and discuss results with a team of parents and professionals who together must make decisions about the student's education. The adapted physical educator is a valuable member of the IEP planning meeting, and must be in attendance at all IEP meetings concerning students referred to or served by the developmental/adapted physical education program.

The IEP Meeting

The purposes of the IEP meeting are to discuss assessment results, to determine if the student is handicapped and therefore eligible for adapted physical education or other special services, and to design, if necessary, an individualized education program. To meet state regulations, this IEP meeting must usually take place within 30 calendar days of a determination that the student is handicapped and in need of special services. A completed IEP must be in place before the services are to be delivered and must be implemented as soon as possible after the meeting. After the initial meeting, an IEP meeting must be held annually to reexamine the appropriateness of the program and to revise when necessary.

Case Manager

When a student has either been previously determined to be handicapped or has been referred for special education assessment for the first time, a *case manager* will be assigned to the student. The case manager's responsibility is ongoing communication with other team members about the status of due process procedures. Usually the case manager is someone specially trained in the area of the student's primary disability. If a student is learning disabled (LD), a teacher specializing in learning disabilities will be the case manager. An adapted physical education teacher will generally be the case manager only for those students whose primary disability is a physical impairment that interferes solely with physical education. Team members turn to the case manager when the following concerns arise:

1. Due date for completed assessments
2. Time and place of IEP meeting
3. Information needed from parents
4. Written parental permission for assessment and implementation of IEP
5. Names of other team members

Notification of the time and place of the IEP meeting should be given to all team members as far in advance of the meeting as possible.

Other Conferences

Teams sometimes meet before IEP meetings. These preparatory meetings have been called assessment review meetings, preplanning conferences, or pre-IEP meetings. They are designed to review assessment results and sometimes to generate IEP objectives before the team meets with the parents. Such conferences are *contrary to* the intent and guidelines of P.L. 94-142, which states that parents or guardians should be considered *equal members* of the IEP team. No educational decisions or discussions are to be made without the involvement of parents. When the assessments are completed, each tester should have summarized and interpreted the test data and should be prepared to share those findings with the *entire* IEP team, *including parents*. All educational decisions are to be made at the IEP conference with input invited from the parents.

Participants in the IEP Meeting

The IEP team is composed of representatives from various allied professions. The team may include (1) the school nurse, (2) a psychologist, (3) a regular physical education teacher, (4) a speech and language clinician, (5) a physical therapist, (6) an occupational therapist, and (7) other special education personnel. The participants at the IEP conference *must include* (1) a representative from the school to supervise the meeting (e.g., principal), (2) the student's teacher or teachers, (3) one or both parents or guardian, (4) the student, if appropriate, and (5) a team member who performed the assessment (e.g., adapted physical education teacher).

Classroom Teacher

The student's assigned classroom teacher must be in attendance at the IEP meeting. For most students, the teacher will be a "homeroom" or regular classroom teacher. The classroom teacher will be a special education teacher for students who are in self-contained programs. At the IEP meeting, the classroom teacher can share observations of the child's physical functioning in the gym, during recess, and while moving throughout the school day. The teacher may also provide valuable insights into the student's personality, attending behavior, social skills, and work habits.

Physical Education Teacher

At an IEP meeting where results of a developmental/adapted physical education assessment are to be discussed, the student's regular physical education teacher should be present. He or she is probably the person who initiated the referral for assessment. During the meeting, the physical education teacher will share observations of the student's participation in class. Also important at this time is learning about the year's schedule of skills and activities to be taught in the regular physical education program. This information will be helpful in writing IEP goals and objectives that are relevant to participation in the regular class. Through discussions at the IEP meeting, the physical education teacher can learn more about the student's strengths, needs, and unique characteristics. Adapted physical education teachers can foster a greater understanding of their roles, and a greater appreciation and awareness of the needs of students who are handicapped, by making sure that the regular physical education teacher attends IEP meetings.

Therapists

For some students, physical or occupational therapists or both will be participating in the IEP meeting. It is most important for the adapted physical educator to note the comments made by these specialists about a student's functioning. A physical therapist may share the results of an evaluation of the student's physical functioning (e.g., range of motion, muscle tone, muscle strength). Suggestions regarding physical therapy, the use of braces or other adaptive equipment, and some general guidelines about physical programming are important to note and discuss in detail later with the therapist.

An occupational therapist may attend IEP meetings for younger students (usually below third grade), or for students who are severely handicapped. The therapist may share results of an evaluation of a student's functional performance in reflex and re-action development, gross and fine motor skills, developmental landmarks, sensori-motor functioning, self-help skills, neuromuscular functioning, and prevocational skills. Since many of these areas overlap and interact with areas assessed in developmental/adapted physical education, particular attention should be paid to the occupational therapist's results and recommendations.

Special Education Teachers

A special education teacher must be in attendance at the IEP meeting. The special education personnel are those who conduct assessment and those who have been providing special services to the student. Special education teachers may be speech and language clinicians; teachers of the learning disabled; of the mildly, moderately, or severely mentally handicapped; or teachers of children who are physically impaired, preschool handicapped emotionally disturbed, hearing impaired, or visually impaired. These teachers, besides the possibility of being appointed case manager, bring essential information to the other team members. They communicate to the team information about the student's disability, learning style, attention span, affective development, behavior repertoire, motivators, and reinforcers. The adapted physical education teacher would be wise to maintain ongoing communication with the special education teacher about the student's progress.

Parent and Student

The parent or parents (or in some cases the guardians) are required to attend the IEP meeting. If they are not in attendance, the program may not be initiated without their written permission.

Parents can offer interesting and helpful information about their child at the IEP meeting. Descriptions of the student's play behavior in the home, the yard, and the neighborhood help give a clearer picture of the student's physical functioning in the natural living environment. A student who resides in a small one-bedroom high-rise apartment may have less opportunity for gross motor play than the student living in a rambler style house in a sprawling suburban neighborhood. Being aware of how physically active a student is at home can be helpful when planning IEP goals and objectives. The IEP meeting provides an ideal opportunity to give suggestions to parents for enhancing play and motor skills at home.

When appropriate, the student may participate in his or her own IEP meeting. Students in intermediate through secondary grade levels who have the ability to participate in the decision-making process should be attending their IEP meetings. Often the student can provide the most insight into her or his own interests and needs in physical education. Students who assist in setting goals and objectives may also be highly motivated to participate in the developmental/adapted physical education program and to monitor their own progress.

The Principal and Others

Federal law mandates that a representative from the local education agency (LEA) participate in and supervise the IEP meeting. The representative is usually the building principal, although an assistant principal, guidance counselor, or teacher can sometimes be designated instead. The principal's role at the IEP meeting is to guide the decision-making process and to be a liaison between school and parents. The principal can offer a unique perspective on the overall administration and management of the proposed individualized program, as well as assist in the communication process and general operation of the meeting.

For some students, there may be additional participants at the IEP meeting. Family physicians, medical specialists, and child advocates sometimes attend IEP meetings. Only persons who have assessment results to present or contributions to make toward the development of the program should participate in the conference.

Communication During the IEP Meeting

While professionals may be well prepared and knowledgeable about the assessment results they bring to an IEP meeting, effective communication among team members is the key to productive decision making. Professional communication means listening, sharing, and discussing, rather than simply reporting test data. The development of an appropriate, valid IEP is the intent of the IEP conference, and this cannot be accomplished without sound communication and collaborative efforts among team members.

Reviewing Rights

Often overlooked and taken for granted are the specific due process rights of parents. While P.L. 94-142 guarantees parental rights in the education of handicapped children, most states have more specific regulations delineating step-by-step due process procedures. At the beginning of each IEP conference, the case manager or designated staff member should briefly explain and review the rights and due process system for the parent or parents present. This review is not intended to be a legal "reading of the rights" activity, but rather a reminder to everyone present that the parent or guardian has an equal partnership role in the decision-making process.

Sharing Results

Each team member who conducted an assessment of the student must present his or her findings at the IEP conference. Since an IEP conference usually takes place in a limited amount of time, here are some general suggestions for efficient reporting.

General Procedure Used.   Begin the report by presenting a brief review of the assessment procedure and why that procedure was chosen. Before reporting test results, give a brief, positive statement about the student, for example, "I really enjoyed working with Bobby. He was very cooperative." If a standardized fitness test was administered, describe briefly why fitness was measured and with which instrument or method. If no standardized tests were used, explain the uniqueness of the child's handicap and why informal methods were selected instead.

Clarity.   The adapted physical education teacher is often the only expert representing the psychomotor domain. The titles of subtests and the motor terminology may sound like jargon to other team members. When reporting results of tests of "bilateral coordination," "agility," or even "balance," explain briefly what each term means and give examples. Team members may be embarrassed about asking questions, and parents may feel intimidated by new terminology.

Reporting Ranges.   Rather than reporting scores or numbers of any kind, the results of an assessment should be explained descriptively. For example, rather than report that Jamie achieved a score of 17 on balance, or that she was at the 10th percentile, it is more readily understandable to report that, "Jamie's balance skill level is below average for her age." McLoughlin and Lewis (1981) proposed a five-level system for reporting assessment results.

1.   Above average: more than 2 standard deviations above the mean
2.   High average: from 1 to 2 standard deviations above the mean
3.   Average: within 1 standard deviation above or below the mean
4.   Low average: from 1 to 2 standard deviations below the mean
5.   Below average: more than 2 standard deviations below the mean

When using this system, the reporter can simply indicate the desired scores, or age equivalents, with the corresponding levels listed above, if desired. Each statement of assessment results should be a statement about the student's current level of performance. As a current skill status is explained, the above system can be used to report strengths as well as weaknesses. When motor performance in one area seems to be related to performance in another area, indicate the relationship.

Recommendations.   While reporting assessment results, postpone making recommendations until later in the conference. As results are summarized and explained, emphasize clearly the areas of strengths and difficulties. It is both professional and wise to listen to the reports of other team members, to ask relevant questions, and to answer the questions that others may have before making recommendations.

Listening to Team Members.   Although the role of the adapted physical education teacher may appear to be one of reporting assessment results and making recommendations, assuming the role of listener is equally important. Parents can provide interesting insights into the student's motor behavior, and personnel such as the school nurse may well have worthwhile observations. Listening to the reports of the special education teachers is crucial, for they can shed light on the student's handicapping condition and unique learning style. Everyone present at the IEP conference plays an important role in shaping the student's education. Listening to each other is what makes the conference work.

Writing the Individualized Education Program (IEP)

Federal mandates are clear about the contents of the IEP (P.L. 94-142, 1977). Each program must include the following:

1. Statement of the student's present levels of educational performance
2. Statement of annual goals, including short-term objectives
3. Statement of the specific educational and related services to be provided to the student, and the extent to which the student will be able to participate in regular educational programs
4. Projected dates for initiation of services and anticipated duration of services
5. Appropriate objective criteria, evaluation procedures, and schedules for determining on at least an annual basis whether the objectives are being achieved

The adapted physical educator who is participating in the development of an IEP plays an active role in writing the program.

Current Level of Performance

The adapted physical education teacher must develop a brief statement about the student's current level of performance in physical education. The statement should indicate general areas of strength as well as weakness in motor skill performance. Depending on the particular format of the IEP, this statement about the current level of performance may be incorporated with statements from other team members.

Annual Goals

Annual goals can be thought of as statements representing skill needs in broad areas. They are statements indicating what is to be achieved within the next year. Annual goals differ greatly from student to student and are based on the student's age, disability, areas of need, and expectations within the regular class. They are determined by examining the subtest areas of poor performance.

Fitness Goals. While physical fitness is a goal for all individuals, it should be listed as an annual goal only for students with significant fitness problems. Physical fitness becomes a more crucial goal for intermediate and secondary grade students than for preschool and primary grade students. Examples of physical fitness annual goals are

1. John will improve abdominal strength.
2. John will improve heart and lung endurance by increasing distance and speed while jogging regularly.
3. John will increase his number of full push-ups by 20 percent.
4. John will improve hip flexibility by increasing distance in the "sit and reach."

Goals of improved physical fitness may include goals involving strength, muscular endurance, cardiovascular endurance, and flexibility.

Locomotor Skill Goals.   For some students at preschool and primary grade levels and for students who are severely handicapped, goals may be needed in the area of locomotion. If a test has revealed difficulties in bilateral coordination and if observations substantiate that locomotor skills are delayed, goals may be written for improving locomotor skills. Sample annual goals for locomotor skills are

1. Beth will demonstrate a mature horizontal jumping pattern in 8 to 10 jumps.
2. Beth will walk unassisted and maintain balance for 10 steps.
3. Beth will demonstrate arm opposition while running.

Locomotor skill goals include creeping, crawling, walking, running, vertical jumping, horizontal jumping, hopping, galloping, skipping, sliding, and leaping. Specially designed locomotion goals may include propelling a wheelchair, or walking with canes or other assistive devices.

Goals for Object Control Skills.   The ability to move while controlling an object is important from preschool through secondary grades. Fundamental skills at the primary grade level form the prerequisite skills for many sports and recreational activities. Sample annual goals for object control skills are

1. Jason will demonstrate a mature overhand throw with distance (30 feet) and accuracy (10-foot diameter target).
2. Jason will grasp a 4-inch nerf ball 9 to 10 times.
3. Jason will demonstrate a functional underhand volleyball serve.
4. Jason will toe-kick a 10-inch playground ball for a distance of 20 feet, 4 to 5 times.

Results on tests of upper-limb coordination, eye-hand coordination, or observations in physical education may generate IEP annual goals in object control skills. Object control skill goals for preschool-age children may include push, pull, reach, grasp, release, and underhand roll. Elementary level skills include overhand throw, catch, kick, batting, underhand strike, and ball bounce. Object control skills at secondary levels include dribbling, shooting baskets, chest pass, one-hand catch, tennis serve, tennis volley, volleyball serve and volley, soccer kicks, soccer dribbling, golf swing, shuffleboard push, racquetball swing, and bowling swing.

Body Management Goals.   Many motor ability tests include subtests that measure the body management components of static and dynamic balance. Goals for improving balance may be appropriate for children at preschool through secondary levels. The challenge to the adapted physical education teacher is to attempt to generalize the results of test items that evaluate balance into meaningful instructional goals and activities. Examples of annual goals in balance include

1. Mary will maintain a 1-foot balance for 10 seconds.
2. Mary will balance on 3 parts of her body for 10 seconds.
3. Mary will walk heel-to-toe for 6 consecutive steps following a 2-inch tape line.
4. Mary will maintain a tripod position for 10 seconds.

Tests that address equilibrium, vestibular system function, or righting reflexes are in essence purporting to measure various factors in the balance domain. Balance items generally are either static (maintaining balance while stationary) or dynamic (maintaining balance while moving).

Other body management goals focus on the areas of agility, spatial direction, body actions, body awareness, and spatial relations. Examples of body management goals are

1. Dan will identify basic body parts on request (body awareness).
2. Dan will move on request according to the directions forward, backward, sideways, up, down, over, and under (spatial direction).
3. Dan will demonstrate the body actions of twist, turn, bend, straighten, and reach on request (body actions).
4. Dan will participate in a large-group physical activity and maintain his own space while respecting the space of others. He will not bump into other children and will watch where he is going (spatial relations).

Body management goals are crucial for preschool and primary grade students, because these goals are building blocks for group activities in physical education.

Goals for Social Skills in Physical Education. An often overlooked area that is essential to safe and successful participation in physical education is social skills. Although the social domain is not considered a part of physical education pursuant to P.L. 94-142, we address social goals here because, mandate or no mandate, social skills are critical in physical education. Some students have movement skills that are acceptable, but demonstrate problems with cooperation, communication, and competition with peers. Difficulties with social skills generally will not be revealed in the results of standardized physical education or motor tests. Social participation is usually assessed by means of recording observed social behaviors during a natural physical education setting. When social problems are clearly interfering with safe and successful participation in physical education, annual social skill goals in the physical education domain should be written into the IEP. Sample annual goals in the social domain are

1. Joe will cooperate with others in gym class by taking turns.
2. Joe will attend physical education class regularly and promptly, except for excused absences.
3. Joe will respect physical education equipment by using it properly and safely.

4. Joe will participate in competitive team games by congratulating the opposing team when his team loses.
5. Joe will listen and follow the teacher's directions in physical education class.

Goals in the social domain may interact with other annual goals of the IEP. When appropriate, goals should be written to include behaviors in more than just the physical education setting. Examples of goals for the social domain include taking turns, decreasing inappropriate behaviors, respecting the performance of others, using equipment properly, accepting competition positively, and improving attending behaviors.

Other Annual Goals.   Annual goals may be written for any problem area in the psychomotor domain. Goals should cover a broad category of skills for which specific objectives are written. Because the IEP is in part a communication tool for the school and the student's parents, annual goals should be written clearly and simply with input from the other team members.

Instructional Objectives and Criteria

Once the annual goals are established delineating major areas of physical education for individualized intervention, specific instructional objectives must be developed for each annual goal area. Instructional, short-term objectives are statements about specific physical education skills to be developed to attain a particular annual goal. For example,

1. *Goal:* To develop a mature running pattern
    Objectives:
    a. Given 1 minute, a running course of at least 50 yards, and the verbal cue, "Run until I say stop," the student will demonstrate running with arms in opposition to legs 90 percent of the time.
    b. Given 1 minute, a running course of at least 50 yards, and the verbal cue, "Run until I say stop," the student will demonstrate running with heel-toe placement 95 percent of the time.
2. *Goal:* To improve abdominal strength
    Objectives:
    a. Given 30 seconds, the student will demonstrate 20 curl-ups with knees bent and hands behind head.
    b. Given 20 seconds, the student will demonstrate continuous V kicks 1 inch from floor while balanced on seat and elbows.
3. *Goal:* To demonstrate a functional vertical jump
    Objectives:
    a. Given a 3-foot square, the student will demonstrate 9 or 10 vertical jumps with feet together, full arm swing, and maintaining balance when landing.

A list of additional sample IEP objectives is included in Appendix B.

When writing instructional objectives, keep in mind the following guidelines:

1. State the motor skill in *behavioral* terms, including positioning (e.g., 30-to-40-degree curl-ups with bent knees and hands clasped behind head).
2. Describe the "givens," the instructional cues, environmental boundaries, time limits, and equipment.
3. State the criteria for attainment, the standard against which the student will be measured (e.g., 9 of 10 trials).

Clarity helps communicate the objectives to parents, team members, and the student, and also provides clear guidelines for teaching and progress evaluation.

Service Delivery

When assessment is completed and student needs identified, the means for meeting the instructional activities must be decided. The program should be determined by individual student needs rather than defining the needs to accommodate the available program facilities. The convenience of facilities, equipment, and programs too often dictate how service to the student is delivered.

Least Restrictive Environment

The student's program should be delivered in the least restrictive environment that meets his or her needs. Figure 2.3 shows the range of adapted physical education services possible. For most students, the provision of developmental/adapted physical education services in the regular physical education class is the least restrictive environment that should be explored. Simple modifications of the regular program and consultation with the regular physical education teacher may be all that are necessary for safe and successful physical education for many students needing developmental/adapted physical education services. For students who are severely handicapped, a completely segregated physical education program conducted on a one-to-one or small-group basis may be the least restrictive environment feasible.

References

McLoughlin, J. A., and Lewis, R. B. *Assessing Special Students*. Columbus, OH: Charles E. Merrill, 1981.

Public Law 94-142, Education for All Handicapped Children Act. *Federal Register* 42(163), August 23, 1977.

Wessel, J. A., Project Director. *I CAN: Primary Skills*. Northbrook, IL: Hubbard, 1976.

Wessel, J. A., Project Director. *I CAN: Sport, Leisure and Recreation Skills*. Northbrook. IL: Hubbard, 1980.

APPENDIX A

Selected Instruments for Adapted Physical Education Assessment

Name of Test and Year	Source	Brief Description of Test
AAHPERD Youth Fitness Test for the Mildly Mentally Retarded (1976)	AAHPERD Publication Sales 1900 Association Drive Reston, VA 22091	A test battery designed for use with mildly MR children is composed of 7 items to evaluate specific aspects of motor performance. Together the items give an overall picture of general levels of physical fitness.
Bayley Scales of Motor Development (1969)	Bayley, N. *Manual for the Bayley Scales of Infant Development.* New York: The Psychological Corporation.	Individually administered test to assess status of children 2 months to $2^{1}/_{2}$ years. Used in recognition and diagnosis of sensory-neurological defects and emotional disturbances.
Body Image Screening Test for Blind Children (1971)	American Foundation for the Blind 15 W. 16th Street New York, NY 10011	
Bruininks-Oseretsky Test of Motor Proficiency (1978)	American Guidance Service Circle Pines, MN 55014	Individually administered test to assess motor functioning. Complete battery, 8 subtests comprised of 46 separate items, provides a comprehensive index of motor proficiency as well as separate measures of gross to fine motor skills.
Cratty Six-Category Gross Motor Test (1969)	Charles C Thomas, Publisher 301-27 E. Lawrence Avenue Springfield, IL 62717	Screening test for perceptual motor functioning.
Denver Developmental Screening Test (1975)	W. K. Frankenburg and J. B. Dodds LADOCA Project Publishing Foundation, Inc. East 51st Ave. and Lincoln St. Denver, CO 80216	A method of screening for evidence of slow development in infants and preschool children.

| Designed for Ages, Disabilities | Standardization Sample | | List of Subtests |
	Size	Population Age Range	
8 to 18 yrs, mildly retarded	4200	Mildly mentally retarded	Arm-shoulder-girdle strength Efficiency of abdominal and hip flexor muscles Speed and agility Explosive muscle power Skill and coordination Cardiovascular efficiency
2 months to 2 yrs, general population	1262	Normal 2 to 30 mos	81 items of gross and fine motor abilities
8 to 19 yrs, blind children (With a few adaptations, the test can be used with sighted, retarded, and deaf children.)	91	Mean age 10.06 yrs	Body planes Body parts Body movements Laterality Directionality
$4^1/_2$ to $14^1/_2$ yrs, general population, including children with disabilities	Two samples used: 250 75	5 to 14 yrs	Static balance Performance balance Coordinated movements Strength Visual motor coordination Response speed Visual motor control Upper-limb speed and precision
4 to 16 yrs ("normal" children) 5 to 20 yrs (E.M.R.)* 5 to 24 yrs (T.M.R.)† 5 to 22 yrs (Down's syndrome)	200		Body perception Gross ability Balance Locomotor Ball throwing Ball tracking
2 wks to 6 yrs, children with delayed development	1036	2 wks to 6 yrs	Gross motor functions Language Fine motor-adaptive Personal-social

Appendix A (continued)

Name of Test and Year	Source	Brief Description of Test
DeOreo: Fundamental Motor Skills Inventory (1976)	Unpublished Kent State University	The DeOreo developmental assessment instrument for use with preschool children examines performance in 11 categories.
Fait Physical Fitness Battery for Mentally Retarded Children (1972)	W. B. Saunders West Washington Square Philadelphia, PA 19105	Measurement of physical fitness.
Fleischman Basic Fitness Test (1964)	Prentice-Hall Englewood Cliffs, NJ 07632	Measurement of physical fitness.
Frostig Developmental Test of Visual Perception (1963)	Consulting Psychologist Press, Inc. 577 College Avenue Palo Alto, CA 94306	Screening device for nursery school, kindergarten, and first grade children or clinical evaluative instrument for older children who exhibit learning disabilities.
Gesell Developmental Schedules (1949)	Gesell, A., and C. S. Amatruda. Gesell Developmental Schedules. New York: Psychological Company.	The schedules are used predominantly in follow-up on infants with complications at birth, or as predictors of intellectual development in preschool and early school years.
Godfrey-Kephart Movement Pattern Checklist (1969)	Appleton-Century-Crofts 292 Madison Avenue New York, NY 10017	Checklist used as screening device for motor development and ability.

| Designed for Ages, Disabilities | Standardization Sample | | List of Subtests |
	Size	Population Age Range	
Preschool, general population	Not available		Striking　Catching Balance　Running Skipping　Climbing Jumping　Throwing Galloping　Kicking Hopping
9 to 20 yrs, E.M.R.,* T.M.R.†		Moderately and mildly M.R. 9 to 20 yrs	Speed Aquatic muscular endurance Dynamic muscular endurance Balance-static Agility Cardio-respiratory endurance
No limit	20,000	12 to 18 yrs	Extent flexibility Dynamic flexibility Explosive strength Static strength Dynamic strength Gross body equilibrium Stamina
4 to 8 yrs, general population	2100	Nursery and public school children	Eye-motor coordination Figure ground Constancy of shape Perception of position in space Perception of spatial relationship
4 wks to 6 yrs			Motor Adaptive Language Personal and social
"Typical and atypical" children			Movement patterns

*E.M.R. = educable mentally retarded
†T.M.R. = trainable mentally retarded

Appendix A (continued)

Name of Test and Year	Source	Brief Description of Test
I CAN Program (1976)	J. A. Wessel Project Director *I CAN:* Primary Skills Hubbard Scientific Co. Northbrook, IL 60062	A developmental physical education program. Sequenced materials include performance objectives, assessment standards, instructional techniques, data forms, and games that reinforce the instructional program.
Lincoln/Oseretsky Motor Development Scale (1955)	C. H. Stoelting Co. 424 N. Homan Avenue Chicago, IL 60624	Motor development test with 36 items designed for use by relatively untrained examiners to assess motor development of children 5–15 years old.
McCarthy Screening Test (1978)	The Psychological Corp. 757 Third Avenue New York, NY 10017	Designed to identify children who may be developmentally lagging, the test assesses performance in cognitive and sensorimotor domains.
Ohio State University Scale of Intra-Gross Motor Assessment (SIGMA) (1975)	Loovis, E. M., Doctoral dissertation, The Ohio State University, University Microfilms #76-3485.	The O.S.U. SIGMA was designed to assess efficiency and maturity of children preschool through 14 yrs in performing 11 selected gross motor skills.
Oregon Data-Based Physical Education Program (1980)	John M. Dunn Dept. of Physical Education Oregon State University Corvallis, OR 97331	Oregon State University, Dept. of Physical Education in cooperation with Teaching Research has developed a data-based physical education program for moderately and severely handicapped students. Information is provided to help teachers place, baseline, implement, and posttest children to determine learning outcomes.
Peabody Developmental Motor Scales (1983)	George Peabody College P.O. Box 163 Nashville, TN 37203	Scales designed as indicators of gross and fine motor skills occurring in children between 0 and 7 yrs.

Designed for Ages, Disabilities	Standardization Sample		List of Subtests	
	Size	Population Age Range		
Preschool (2 to 5 yrs), Primary (5 to 14 yrs), Secondary (15 to 25 yrs), general handicapped or nonhandicapped			Aquatics Body management Health and fitness Fundamental skills Preschool skills Team sports Dance and individual sports Backyard/neighborhood activities Outdoor activities	
6 to 14 yrs	380 males 362 females	6 to 14 yrs	Hand and arm movements Gross motor	
$4^{1}/_{2}$ to 6 yrs, developmentally lagging			Right left orientation Verbal memory Draw a design Numerical memory Conceptual grouping Leg coordination	
Preschool through 14 yrs, general population	12	2 to 14 yrs	Walking Catching Ladder climbing Stair climbing Throwing Striking Skipping	Running Hopping Jumping Kicking
Severely handicapped			Movement concepts Elementary games Physical fitness skills Lifetime leisure skills	
0 to 7 yrs, general population			Gross motor Fine motor	

Appendix A (continued)

Name of Test and Year	Source	Brief Description of Test
Portage Project	Deborah Cochran, Project Director Portage Project CESA 12 P.O. Box 564 Portage, WI 53901	Developmentally formulated program for children 0 to 6 yrs. The project is designed to improve adjustments of a child at school and at home. Portage comes in three parts: (1) checklist of behaviors, (2) color code file listing possible teaching methods, (3) manual of directions.
Project A.C.T.I.V.E.: Basic Motor Ability Test		Project A.C.T.I.V.E. is a comprehensive adapted physical education program. Materials available to assist teachers provide appropriate physical education for children with a wide range of disabilities.
Project Unique: The Physical Fitness and Performance of Sensory and Orthopedically Impaired Youth (1979)	State University of New York College at Brockport Brockport, NY 14420	A three-year federally funded project designed to study and establish normative data for sensory and orthopedically handicapped children, ages 10–17, throughout the U.S.
Purdue Perceptual Motor Survey (1966)	Roach, Eugene G., and Newell C. Kephart. *The Purdue Perceptual-Motor Survey.* Columbus, OH: Charles E. Merrill, 1966.	A survey that allows the practitioner to observe a broad spectrum of behavior in a structured, but not stereotyped, set of circumstances.
Rarick-Factor Structure of Motor Abilities of Trainable Mentally Retarded Children (1977)	Unpublished. G. Lawrence Rarick Dept. of Physical Education U. of California Berkeley, CA 94720	A 7-item test that measures motor proficiency of trainable mentally retarded children.
Southern California Sensory Integration Test (1976)	Western Psychological Services, Publishers and Distributors 12031 Wilshire Blvd. Los Angeles, CA 90025	Intended to measure sensory integrative dysfunction in underlying neural systems, thought to accompany learning problems.

| Designed for Ages, Disabilities | Standardization Sample | | List of Subtests |
	Size	Population Age Range	
0 to 6 yrs, general population			Cognitive Self help Motor Language Socialization
Prekindergarten through adult, normal, mentally retarded, learning disabled, and emotionally disturbed			Gross body coordination Balance/postural orientation Eye/hand coordination Eye/hand accuracy Eye/foot accuracy
10 to 17 yrs, sensory and orthopedically handicapped			Body composition Dynamic strength and endurance Agility Static balance Flexibility Static muscular strength Explosive muscle strength Cardio-respiratory function
No age limit, mentally retarded	200	6 to 10 yrs	Balance and posture Body image and differentiation Perceptual motor match Ocular control Form perception
Norms provided for 6 to 21 yrs, trainable mentally retarded			7 items
3 yrs to adult, perceptual difficulties	Variable, but small (e.g., n = 30)	Unspecified	17 subtests (e.g., space visualization, F-G perception, kinesthesia, manual form perception, finger identification, graphethesia, motor accuracy)

Appendix A (continued)

Name of Test and Year	Source	Brief Description of Test
Stott's Test of Motor Impairment (1972)	Brook Educational Publishing Ltd. Box 1171 Guelph, Ontario	Assess and ascertain motor impairment of functional or presumed neurological origin.
Texas Revision of Fait's Basic Motor Skill Test (1978)	Fait, Hollis F. *Special Physical Education: Adapted, Corrective, Developmental.* Philadelphia: W. B. Saunders, 1978, pp. 76–77.	The test measures specific motor skills judged most needed by handicapped children to function efficiently in everyday life. Twenty skills are assessed including walking, pushing, ascending and descending stairs, and jumping.
Vineland Adaptation of Oseretsky Test (1949)		

| Designed for Ages, Disabilities | Standardization Sample | | List of Subtests |
	Size	Population Age Range	
5 to 16 yrs			Control and balance of the body while immobile Control and coordination of the upper limbs Control and coordination of the body while in motion Manual dexterity Simultaneous movement/precision
Mentally deficient children	100		Static coordination Dynamic manual coordination of hands General dynamic coordination Motor speed Simultaneous movement

APPENDIX B

Sample Individualized Education Program Objectives

Sample 1
Physical Fitness Objectives

1. The student will demonstrate arm-shoulder strength by executing a "seal walk" with straight arms, dragging straight legs with ankles crossed, for a distance of 15 feet.
2. Given a 7-inch nerf ball on side table at waist height, the student will complete 10 consecutive nerf ball "presses" with each arm, while sitting in his or her wheelchair, to improve tricep strength.
3. The student will demonstrate 5 forward "windmills" and 5 backward "windmills" using full shoulder rotation.
4. The student will demonstrate improved heart-lung endurance by increasing time using the exercycle to 20 minutes daily.
5. The student will increase the number of balloons blown up in 10 minutes to 10 balloons.

Sample 2
Locomotor Objectives

1. The student will efficiently wheel her wheelchair through an obstacle course, executing turns, stops, and starts as instructed.
2. The student will demonstrate a mature walking pattern with a sighted guide.
3. The student will demonstrate improved agility (turns, starts, and stops) in regular physical education while wearing his leg prosthesis during classes.
4. Given the verbal cue "Come here," the student will crawl, using forearms with head up, forward 6 feet to an object.
5. Given a starting line and the cue "Jump," the student will demonstrate a mature horizontal jump 3 out of 5 times.
6. The student will demonstrate 10 consecutive "double-jumps" on a long jump rope.

Sample 3
Object Control Objectives

1. Given a basketball, the student will demonstrate mature ball dribbling with both the dominant and nondominant hands (individually) continuously for 30 seconds.
2. Given a basketball, the student will demonstrate a functional chest pass 9 out of 10 times.
3. Given a 10-inch balloon, the student will keep it in the air by continuous taps for 30 seconds.
4. Given a 10-inch nerf ball thrown at various heights, the student will demonstrate a mature catch and appropriate movement into position.

Index

Student Survey

Judy K. Werder and Leonard H. Kalakian
ASSESSMENT IN ADAPTED PHYSICAL EDUCATION

Students, send us your ideas!

The authors and the publisher want to know how well this book served you and what can be done to improve it for those who will use it in the future. By completing and returning this questionnaire, you can help us develop better textbooks. We value your opinion and want to hear your comments. Thank you.

Your name (optional) _____ School _____

Your mailing address _____

City _____ State _____ ZIP _____

Instructor's name (optional) _____ Course title _____

1. How does this book compare with other texts you have used? (Check one)
   ☐ Superior   ☐ Better than most   ☐ Comparable   ☐ Not as good as most

2. Circle those chapters you especially liked:
   Chapters: 1 2 3 4 5 6 7
   Comments:

3. Circle those chapters you think could be improved:
   Chapters: 1 2 3 4 5 6 7
   Comments:

4. Please rate the following. (Check one for each line)

	Excellent	Good	Average	Poor
Readability of text material	( )	( )	( )	( )
Logical organization	( )	( )	( )	( )
General layout and design	( )	( )	( )	( )
Up-to-date treatment of subject	( )	( )	( )	( )
Match with instructor's course organization	( )	( )	( )	( )
Illustrations that clarify the text	( )	( )	( )	( )
Selection of topics	( )	( )	( )	( )
Explanation of difficult concepts	( )	( )	( )	( )

(Over, please)

5. List any chapters that your instructor did not assign. _____

_____

6. What additional topics did your instructor discuss that were not covered in the text? _____

_____

7. Did you buy this book new or used?   ☐New   ☐Used
   Do you plan to keep the book or sell it?   ☐Keep it   ☐Sell it
   Do you think your instructor should continue
   to assign this book?   ☐Yes   ☐No

8. After taking the course, are you interested in taking more courses in this field?
   ☐Yes   ☐No
   Did you take this course to fulfill a requirement, or as an elective?
   ☐Required   ☐Elective

9. What is your major? _____
   Your class rank?   ☐Freshman ☐Sophomore ☐Junior ☐Senior ☐Other, specify:

10. GENERAL COMMENTS:

May we quote you in our advertising?   ☐Yes   ☐No

Please remove this page and mail to: Mary L. Paulson
                                            Burgess Publishing Company
                                            7108 Ohms Lane
                                            Minneapolis, MN 55435

THANK YOU!